Ernst Schering Research Foundation Workshop
Supplement 11
Regenerative and Cell Therapy

Ernst Schering Research Foundation Workshop
Supplement 11

Regenerative and Cell Therapy

Clinical Advances

A. Keating, K. Dicke, N. Gorin, R. Weber, H. Graf
Editors

With 13 Figures

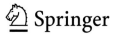 Springer

Series Editors: G. Stock and M. Lessl

Library of Congress Control Number: 2004105981

ISSN 1431-7133
ISBN 3-540-22093-3 Springer Berlin Heidelberg New York

Springer is a part of Springer Science+Business Media
springeronline.com

© Springer-Verlag Berlin Heidelberg 2005
Printed in Germany

Editor: Dr. Ute Heilmann, Heidelberg
Desk editor: Wilma McHugh, Heidelberg
Production editor: Andreas Gösling, Heidelberg
Cover design: design & production GmbH, Heidelberg
Typesetting: K+V Fotosatz GmbH, Beerfelden

Printed on acid-free paper – 21/3130/AG-5 4 3 2 1 0

Preface

Clinical success in hematopoietic stem cell transplantation have paved the way into the new world of regenerative medicine. Open issues important for the translation of scientific achievements into therapeutic strategies have been debated on different levels: stem cell biology, manufacturing and clinical use.

In the face of all ongoing laboratory research, investigators have proceeded, some quietly, some with fanfare to conduct clinical trials of cell therapy for a wide variety of human ailments.

This book, inspired by a symposium on regenerative and cell therapy held at the Sorbonne in Paris in 2003, attempts to evaluate the clinical advances in this area in the context of earlier or contemporaneous research with in vitro and animal models as well as preclinical studies.

We believe that an evaluation of clinical progress in cell therapy is timely, may help to identify issues that require more preclinical investigation before proceeding to clinical trials, or importantly, identify areas that are ripe for further immediate clinical intervention. Similarly, bedside to bench issues may become more readily apparent and may foster the investigative loop that occasionally moves clinical development rapidly to the next level. The juxtaposition of regenerative cell therapy, especially for damaged myocardium, with the longer established clinical experience in anticancer cell therapy, such as allotransplantation and adoptive immunotherapy, is deliberate – we hope that mutually instructive insights will arise.

Finally, we are most grateful to all the authors, who are international leaders in the field, for their thoughtful contributions.

Armand Keating
On behalf of coeditors *Karel Dicke, Norbert Gorin, Renate Weber,* and *Hermann Graf.*

Contents

List of Editors and Contributors

Editors

Keating, A.
Princess Margaret Hospital, Ontario Cancer Institute, Toronto,
Ontario, Canada
e-mail: armand.keating@uhn.on.ca

Coeditors

Dicke, K.
Arlington Cancer Center, Arlington, TX, USA
e-mail: kdicke@acctx.com

Gorin, N.
Hospital Saint-Antoine, Paris, France
e-mail: norbert-claude.gorin@sat.ap-hop-paris.fr

Weber, R.
Schering AG, Müllerstr. 178, 13342 Berlin, Germany
e-mail: renate.weber@schering.de

Graf, H.
Schering AG, Müllerstr. 178, 13342 Berlin, Germany
e-mail: hermann.graf@schering.de

Contributors

Atala, A.
Wake Forest University School of Medicine, Department of Urology,
Medical Center Boulevard, Winston Salem, NC 27157, USA
e-mail: a.atala@tch.harvard.edu

Bollard, C.
Center for Cell and Gene Therapy, Baylor College of Medicine,
The Methodist Hospital and Texas Children's Hospital, Houston,
TX 77030, USA
e-mail: cmbollar@txccc.org

Brenner, M. K.
Section of Hematology-Oncology, Baylor College of Medicine,
Center for Cell and Gene Therapy, 6621 Fannin Street, 3-3320,
Houston, TX 77030-2303, USA
e-mail: mbrenner@bcm.tmc.edu

Cossu, G.
Stem Cell Research Institute, Via Olgettina 58, 20132 Milan, Italy
e-mail: cossu.giulio@hsr.it

Douay, L.
Hôpital d'Enfants, Armand-Trousseau, 26 Avenue du Docteur
A. Netter, Cedex 12, 75571 Paris, France
e-mail: luc.douay@trs.ap-hop-paris.fr

Fitzpatrick, L. A.
Endocrine Research Unit, Department of Endocrinology, Diabetes,
Metabolism, Nutrition and Internal Medicine, Mayo Clinic,
200 First Street SW, Rochester, MN 55905, USA
e-mail: fitz@mayo.edu

Fouillard, L.
Service des Maladies du Sang, Hôpital Saint Antoine,
184 rue du Faubourg Saint Antoine, 75012 Paris, France
e-mail: fouillar@ext.jussieu.fr

Gordon, P. L.
Divisions of Stem Cell Transplantation and Experimental
Hematology, St. Jude Children's Research Hospital,
332 N. Lauderdale, Memphis, TN 38105, USA
e-mail: patricia.gordon@stjude.org

Heslop, H. E.
Baylor College of Medicine, Center for Cell and Gene Therapy,
6621 Fannin Street, 3-3320, Houston, TX 77030-2303, USA
e-mail: hheslop@bcm.tmc.edu

Horwitz, E. M.
Divisions of Stem Cell Transplantation and Experimental
Hematology, St. Jude Children's Research Hospital,
332 N. Lauderdale, Memphis, TN 38105, USA
e-mail: Edwin.horwitz@stjude.org

Huls, M. H.
Baylor College of Medicine, Center for Cell and Gene Therapy,
6621 Fannin Street, 3-3320, Houston, TX 77030-2303, USA
e-mail: hhuls@bcm.tmc.edu

Koh, C. J.
Institute for Regenerative Medicine, Wake Forest University School
of Medicine, Medical Center Blvd, Winston Salem, NC 27157, USA
e-mail: c.koh@tch.harvard.edu

Koo, W. W. K.
Wayne State University, Detroit, Michigan, USA
e-mail: wkoo@wayne.edu

Kurbegov, D.
MD Anderson Cancer Center, 1515 Holcome Boulevard, Houston,
TX 77030, USA
e-mail: dkurbego@mail.mdanderson.org

Menasché, P.
Service de Chirurgie Cardio Vasculaire, Hôpital Bichat, 46 rue Henri
Huchard, 75018 Paris, France
e-mail: philippe.menasche@bch.ap-hop-paris.fr

Molldrem, J.
MD Anderson Cancer Center, 1515 Holcome Boulevard, Houston,
TX 77030, USA
e-mail: jmolldre@mail.mdanderson.org

Neel, M. D.
Divisions of Stem Cell Transplantation and Experimental
Hematology, St. Jude Children's Research Hospital,
332 N. Lauderdale, Memphis, TN 38105, USA
e-mail: mneel@wnm.net

Rooney, C. M.
Baylor College of Medicine, Center for Cell and Gene Therapy,
6621 Fannin Street, 3-3320, Houston, TX 77030-2303, USA
e-mail: crooney@bcm.tmc.edu

Schwartz, M.
Department of Neurobiology, Building for Brain Research,
Weizmann Institute of Science, P.O. Box 26, Rehovot 76100, Israel
e-mail: michal.Schwartz@weizmann.ac.il

Storb, R.
Fred Hutchinson Cancer Research Center, 1100 Fairview Avenue
North, D1-100, P.O. Box 19024, Seattle, WA 98109-1024, USA
e-mail: rstorb@fhcrc.org

1 Problems and Hopes with Cell Therapy: The Case of Muscular Dystrophy

G. Cossu

1.1 Introduction

In muscular dystrophies skeletal muscle fibers progressively degenerate. Lack of one of several proteins located either at the plasma membrane (Blake et al. 2002) or, less frequently, within internal membranes (Nishino and Ozawa 2002) increases the probability of damage during contraction and eventually leads to fiber degeneration, although the molecular mechanisms are not yet understood in detail (Burton and Davies 2002; Emery 2002). Fiber degeneration is counteracted by regeneration of new fibers at the expense of resident

myogenic cells, located underneath the basal lamina and termed satellite cells (Mauro 1961). Although satellite cells were considered
the only cell endowed with myogenic potential (Bischoff 1994), evidence has accumulated showing that other progenitor cells may participate in muscle regeneration (Seale et al. 2001). These latter cells
are probably derived from distinct anatomical sites, such as the microvascular niche of the bone marrow, and reach skeletal muscle
through the circulation and possibly with the incoming vessels.
Balance between fiber degeneration and regeneration dictates the
cellular and clinical outcome. In the most severe forms, such as
Duchenne muscular dystrophy, regeneration is exhausted and skeletal muscle is progressively replaced by fat and fibrous tissue. This
condition leads the patient to progressive weakness and eventually
death by respiratory and/or cardiac failure.

Current therapeutic approaches, mainly represented by steroids,
result in modest beneficial effects (Skuka et al. 2002). Novel experimental approaches (Cossu and Clemens 2001) can be schematically
grouped in three major areas: (a) gene therapy aiming at the production of new viral vectors (mainly adeno, adeno-associated, lenti, and
herpes vectors) less antigenic and more efficient in transducing adult
muscle fibers, (b) novel pharmacological approaches, focusing on
high-throughput screens for molecules that may interfere with patho-
genetic pathways. The search should hopefully identify molecules
that cause skipping of the mutated exon (De Angelis et al. 2002) or
upregulate utrophin synthesis, a cognate protein that compensates for
dystrophin absence when overexpressed in dystrophic mice (Deconinck et al. 1997), (c) cell therapy, based initially on myoblast transplantation and, more recently on the transplantation of stem/progeni-
tor cells. The recent identification of novel types of stem cells opens
new perspectives for cell therapy, the topic of this chapter; however,
the limited knowledge of stem cell biology still represents an obsta-
cle that must be overcome in order to devise protocols with a significant prospect of clinical improvement in patients affected by severe
forms of muscular dystrophy.

1.2 Early Attempts with Myoblasts Transplantation

In 1989, Partridge and his collaborators showed that intramuscular injection of C2C12 cells, an immortal myogenic cell line derived from adult satellite cells, would reconstitute with high efficiency dystrophin positive, apparently normal fibers in dystrophic mdx mice (Partridge et al. 1989). This result caused immediate hopes for therapy and within a few months led to a number of clinical trials in the early 1990s. Myogenic cells were isolated from immune compatible donors, expanded in vitro, and injected in a specific muscle of the patient. These clinical trials failed (for a review see Partridge 1996) due to a number of reasons, some of which may have been predicted (at variance with C2 human myogenic cells do not have unlimited life-span and are not syngeneic between donor and host), while others have become apparent long after the start of the trials. For example, most injected cells (up to 99%) succumb first to an inflammatory response and then to an immune reaction (Beauchamp et al. 1999) against donor cell antigens. Cells that survive do not migrate more than few mm away from the injection site, indicating that innumerable injections should be performed to provide a homogeneous distribution of donor cells. Even though donor myogenic cells can survive for a decade in the injected muscle (Gussoni et al. 1997), the overall efficiency of the process soon made it clear that, although biologically interesting, this approach would have been clinically hopeless.

In the following years, the laboratory of Tremblay has focused on these problems and in a stepwise manner has produced progressive increase in the survival success of injected myoblasts and in their colonization efficiency. Immune-suppression and injection of neutralizing antibodies (directed against surface molecules of infiltrating cells such as LFA1), pretreatment of myoblasts in vitro with growth factors, and modification of the muscle connective tissue all contributed to this improvement (Kinoshita et al. 1994; Guerette et al. 1997). Extension of this protocol to primates (Kinoshita et al. 1996) opens the possibility of a new clinical trial in the near future and with much more information than was available in the trials failed 13 years ago. On a parallel route, several laboratories, including our own, developed strategies to expand in vitro myoblasts from the patients, transduce them with viral vectors encoding the therapeutic gene, and inject them back into a few life essential muscles of the same patients from which they had been initially derived. This approach would solve the problem of donor cell rejection but not of an immune reaction against the vector and the therapeutic gene, a new antigen in genetic diseases. In this case, however, it soon became clear that it was very difficult to produce an integrating vector that would accommodate the very large cDNA of dystrophin. The generation of a microdystrophin (containing both protein ends but missing most of the internal exons) appears to have very recently solved this problem, at least in part (Harper et al. 2002). However, the limited life-span of myogenic cells isolated from dystrophic patients appeared as an even worse problem, and all the attempts to solve it, ranging from immortalization with oncogenes or telomerase to myogenic conversion of nonmyogenic cells, again produced biologically interesting but clinically inadequate results (Decary et al. 1997; Lattanzi et al. 1998; Berghella et al. 1999).

1.3 Why Bone Marrow Transplantation?

The search for cells that may be converted to a myogenic phenotype led us to identify a cryptic myogenic potential in a large number of cells within the mesoderm, including the bone marrow. For these studies we took advantage of a transgenic mouse expressing a nuclear lacZ under the control of muscle-specific regulatory elements (MLC3F-nlacz) only in striated muscle (Kelly et al. 1995). Since direct injection into the muscle tissue is a very inefficient and impractical cell delivery route, bone marrow-derived progenitors immediately appeared as a potential alternative to myoblasts and satellite cells, since they could be systemically delivered to a dystrophic muscle. To test this possibility, we transplanted MLC3F-nlacZ bone marrow into lethally irradiated *scid/bg* mice and, when reconstitution by donor bone marrow had occurred, induced muscle regeneration by cardiotoxin injection into a leg muscle (tibialis *anterior*). Histochemical analysis unequivocally showed the presence of β-gal-staining nuclei at the center and periphery of regenerated fibers, demonstrating for the first time that murine bone marrow contains transplantable progenitors that can be recruited to an injured muscle through the peripheral circulation, and that participate in muscle repair by undergoing differentiation into mature muscle fibers (Ferrari et al. 1998). The publication of this report raised new interest in myogenic progenitors and in their possible clinical use. It was reasoned that, although the frequency of the phenomenon was very low, in a chronically regenerating, dystrophic muscle myogenic progenitors would have found a favorable environment and consequently would have contributed significantly to regeneration of dystrophin positive, normal fibers.

This, however, turned out not to be the case. In the following year, the groups of Kunkel and Mulligan showed that *mdx* mice transplanted with the bone marrow side population (SP) cells [side population cells represent a fraction of total cells that is separated by dye exclusion and contains stem/progenitor cells able to repopulate the hematopoietic system upon transplantation (Goodell et al. 1996)] of syngeneic C57BL/10 mice develop, within several weeks, a small number of dystrophin-positive fibers containing genetically marked (Y chromosome) donor nuclei (Gussoni et al. 1999). Even after many months from the transplantation, the number of fibers carrying both dystrophin and the Y chromosome never exceeded 1% of the total fibers in the average muscle, thus precluding a direct clinical translation for this protocol. Similar results were later obtained in a slightly different animal model, the *mdx4ev* mutant by Ferrari et al. (Ferrari et al. 2001). Very recently, retrospective analysis in a Duchenne patient that had undergone bone marrow transplantation confirmed persistence of donor-derived skeletal muscle cells over a period of many years, again at very low frequency (Gussoni et al. 2002).

Reasons for this low efficiency may be (a) paucity of myogenic progenitors in the bone marrow, (b) inadequate transplantation, a procedure optimized for hematopoietic reconstitution, (c) insufficient signals to recruit myogenic progenitors from the bone marrow, (d) inadequate environment to promote survival, proliferation, and/or differentiation of these progenitors because of competition by resident satellite cells (that sustain regeneration for most of the *mdx* mouse lifespan) or unfavorable environment created by inflammatory cells, (e) difficulties in reaching regenerating fibers because of the increased deposition of fibrous tissue and reduced vascular bed of the dystrophic muscle. Although in dystrophic muscle disease (DMD) patients, regeneration by endogenous satellite cells is exhausted much earlier in life than in the mouse, and therefore muscle colonization by blood-born progenitors may be different, the data by Gussoni et al. (Gussoni et al. 2002) suggests that in any case the process occurs with low frequency.

1.4 Multipotent Stem Cells in the Bone Marrow

Bone marrow hosts a number of multipotent cells, which include hematopoietic stem cells (HSC), mesenchymal stem cells (MSC) and, recently added to the list, multipotent adult progenitors (MAP), endothelial progenitor cells (EPC), and mesoangioblasts (MAB).

These cells are described in detail in different chapters of this book: here we will briefly review their features concerning their myogenic potential and consequently their possible use in preclinical models of muscular dystrophy.

1.4.1 Hematopoietic Stem Cells

Surprisingly, no data are available on the ability of purified HSC to differentiate into skeletal muscle in vitro or in vivo, save the evidence presented by Gussoni et al. of the myogenic potential of the bone marrow SP population, certainly not a pure one. In the case of liver, for example, highly purified HSC were shown to differentiate into hepatocytes (Lagasse et al. 2000). In the case of skeletal muscle, only preliminary and largely unpublished evidence suggest that HSC may have an intrinsic myogenic potential. When bone marrow was fractionated into CD45 positive and negative fractions, the muscle-forming activity was associated with the $CD45^+$ fraction (Ferrari Mavilio 2002); human cord blood CD34 positive cells, after in vitro expansion, differentiate at a significant frequency (5%–10%) into skeletal myotubes when cocultured with murine myoblasts (M. Sampaolesi et al. unpublished observations); circulating human AC133 positive cells also differentiate into skeletal muscles in vitro and in vivo when injected into dystrophic immunodeficient mice (Torrente et al. 2004). Together these data suggest that a myogenic potential is present in the hematopoietic stem cell itself or in a yet-to-be-identified cell that, however, expresses several markers in common with true HSC. If the former were the case, then we would be able to apply a huge amount of knowledge from both experimental and clinical hematology to the design of clinical protocols for muscular dystrophy. Still, additional steps would have to be devised since we already know that bone marrow transplantation is likely to be insufficient to ameliorate the dystrophic phenotype. Specifically, homing of progenitor cells to muscle would have to be stimulated since HSC naturally home to the bone marrow and, equally important, HSC would have to be directed to a myogenic fate with much higher efficiency than what is currently observed. Transient expression of leukocyte adhesion proteins and inducible expression of MyoD may be steps in this direction.

1.4.2 Mesenchymal Stem Cells

Initially identified by Friedenstein et al. (Friedenstein et al. 1966), mesenchymal stem cells mainly originate from perycytes, are located in the perivascular district of the bone marrow stroma and are the natural precursors of bone, cartilage, and fat, the constituent tissues of the bone (Prockop 1997).

Although MSC were reported to give rise to myotubes in culture upon induction with 5 azacytidine (Wakitani et al. 1995), they do not differentiate into muscle under normal conditions (Bianco and Cossu 1999). When transplanted in sheep fetus in utero, human MSC colonized most tissues, including skeletal muscle, although their effective muscle differentiation was not demonstrated (Liechty et al. 2000). Despite the fact that MSC can be easily expanded in vitro, they do not appear at the moment among the best candidates in protocols aimed at reconstituting skeletal muscle in primary myopathies.

1.4.3 Endothelial Progenitor Cells

Initially identified as CD34$^+$, Flk-1$^+$ circulating cells (Asahara et al. 1997), endothelial progenitor cells (EPC) were shown to be transplantable and to participate actively in angiogenesis in a variety of physiological and pathological conditions (Asahara et al. 1999). In vitro expansion of EPC is still problematic and few laboratories have succeeded in optimizing this process. The clear advantage of EPC would be their natural homing to the site of angiogenesis that would target them to the site of muscle regeneration. However, their ability to differentiate into skeletal muscle has not been tested to date.

1.4.4 Multipotent Adult Progenitors

The group of Verfaille (Reyes et al. 2001) has recently identified a rare cell, within mesenchymal stem cell (MSC) cultures from human or rodent (bone marrow) BM, which was termed multipotent adult progenitor cell (MAPC). This cell can be expanded for over 70–150 population doublings (PDs) and differentiates not only into mesenchymal lineage cells but also endothelium, neuroectoderm, and endoderm. Similar cells can be selected from mouse muscle and brain, suggesting that they may be associated with the microvascular niche of probably many if not all tissues of the mammalian body (Jiang et al. 2002 a). Furthermore, when injected into a blastocyst, MAP cells colonize all the tissues of the embryo, with a frequency comparable with ES cells (Jiang et al. 2002 b). Because of their apparently unlimited lifespan and multipotency, MAP cells appear as obvious candidates for many cell replacement therapies, although complete differentiation into the desired cell type still needs to be optimized. As concerns skeletal muscle, neither the frequency at which MAP differentiate into skeletal muscle cells after Azacytidine treatment, nor attempts to optimize this process have been reported. In addition, the ability of MAP to travel through the body using the circulatory route has not been formally demonstrated, although the general features of these cells strongly suggest this to be the case. It will be interesting in the future to see whether MAP cells may restore a normal phenotype in mouse models of muscular dystrophy.

1.4.5 Mesoangioblasts

Searching for the origin of the bone marrow cells that contribute to muscle regeneration (Ferrari et al. 1998) we identified, by clonal analysis, a progenitor cell derived from the embryonic aorta, that shows similar morphology to adult satellite cells and expresses a number of myogenic and endothelial markers also expressed by satellite cells. In vivo aorta-derived myogenic progenitors participate in muscle regeneration and fuse with resident satellite cells (De Angelis et al. 1999). The expression of endothelial markers in satellite cells (VE-cadherin, VEGFR2, etc.) was also unpredicted at the time but later, clonal analysis in vivo by retroviral labeling confirmed the existence of bipotent endothelial skeletal myogenic progenitors in the avian embryos (Kardon et al. 2002). To test the role of these progenitors in vitro we grafted quail or mouse embryonic aorta into host chick embryos. Donor cells, initially incorporated into the host vessels, were later integrated into mesoderm tissues, including bone marrow, cartilage, bone, smooth, skeletal, and cardiac muscle. When expanded on a feeder layer of embryonic fibroblasts, the clonal progeny of a single cell from the mouse dorsal aorta acquired unlimited life-span, expressed hemoangioblastic markers (CD34, Flkl, and c-Kit) and maintained multipotency in culture or when transplanted into a chick embryo. We concluded that these newly identified, vessel-associated stem cells, the meso-angioblasts, participate in postembryonic development of the mesoderm and speculate that postnatal mesodermal stem cells may be rooted in a vascular developmental origin (Minasi et al. 2002).

Inasmuch as mesoangioblasts can be expanded indefinitely, are able to circulate, and are easily transduced with lentiviral vectors, they appeared as a potential novel strategy for the cell therapy of genetic diseases. In principle, mesoangioblasts can be derived from the patient, expanded and transduced in vitro and then reintroduced into the arterial circulation, leading to colonization of the downstream tissues. In recent months we have succeeded in isolating mesoangioblasts from juvenile tissues of the mouse and from human fetal vessels. Attempts to isolate the same cells from postnatal human vessels are in progress at the time of writing.

When injected into the blood circulation, mesoangioblasts accumulate in the first capillary filter they encounter and are able to migrate outside the vessel, but only in the presence of inflammation, as in the case of dystrophic muscle. We thus reasoned that if these cells were injected into an artery, they would accumulate into the capillary filter and from there into the interstitial tissue of downstream muscles. Indeed, intra-arterial delivery of wild-type mesoangioblasts in the a sarcoglycan KO mouse, a model for limb girdle muscular dystrophy (Duclos et al. 1998), corrects morphologically and functionally the dystrophic phenotype of all the muscle downstream of the injected vessel (Sampaolesi et al. 2003). Furthermore, mesoangioblasts, isolated from small vessels of juvenile (P15) a sarcoglycan null mice, were transduced with a lentiviral vector expressing the a sarcoglycan-EGFP fusion protein, injected into the femoral artery of null mice, and reconstituted skeletal muscle similarly to wild-type cells. These data represent the first successful attempt to treat a murine model of limb-girdle myopathy with a novel class of autologous stem cells. Widespread distribution through the capillary network represents the distinct advantage of this strategy over alternative approaches of cell or gene therapy (Sampaolesi et al. 2003).

1.5 Stem Cells with a Myogenic Potential from Tissues Other than Bone Marrow

In the last few years many reports have described the presence of multipotent stem cells in a variety of tissues of the mammalian body. In addition to bone marrow and skeletal muscle, stem cells able to form skeletal muscle have been described in the nervous system (Galli et al. 2000), adipose tissue (Zuk et al. 2001), and in the synovia (De Bari et al. 2003). Although in these reports, evidence for muscle repair in vivo was provided, no data were reported of efficacious amelioration of dystrophic phenotype.

In conclusion, of the many types of stem cells with a myogenic potential (Table 1), only mesoangioblasts have been shown so far to be effective in restoring to a significant extent the dystrophic phenotype in a murine model of dystrophy.

Unfortunately, human mesoangioblasts from patients have not yet been isolated (although preliminary work suggests this to be possible). Several of the other types of stem cells, already isolated from

Table 1. A comparison of different types of mesoderm stem cells with respect to their potential to contribute to muscle regeneration in a dystrophic muscle

Stem cell	Source	Growth in vitro	Crossing muscle endothelium	Myogenic differentiation	Effect in primary myopathies
HSC	BM	Yes	Upon induction	Upon induction	Unknown
MSC	BM	Yo	Unknown	Poor	Unknown
EPC	Microvessels	No	Unknown	Unknown	Unknown
MAP	Bone marrow	Yes	Unknown	Upon induction	Unknown
MAB	Microvessels	Yes	Upon induction	Upon induction	Yes
NSC	Subventricular	Yes	Unknown	Upon induction	Unknown

A schematic and simplified overview of the features, known, presumed, or under scrutiny of different adult stem cells in the perspective of use for cell therapy. Source is generic, since the exact location within bone marrow is uncertain for some stem cells.
HSC, hematopoietic stem cells; MSC, mesenchymal stem cells; EPC, endothelial progenitor cells; MAP, multipotent adult progenitors; MAB, mesoangioblasts; NSC, neural stem cells

adult human tissues, show the potential of achieving similar results, since they can be expanded in vitro, delivered systemically, and induced to differentiate into skeletal muscle. It will be interesting in the future to see which of these different cell types will maintain this promise.

1.6 The Cellular Environment of a Dystrophic Muscle

Before the appearance of stem cells on the scene, the histological situation of a dystrophic muscle could be described with relatively few players (Grounds 1999). Muscle fibers undergo degeneration for the lack of one important protein. This leads to activation of resident satellite cells that proliferate and give rise to myogenic cells that repair damaged fibers or replace dead fibers with new ones. Satellite cells should also give rise to new satellite cells (though this has not yet been formally demonstrated) to ensure a reserve population for further cycles of regeneration: failure of this process, especially in the most severe forms of dystrophy, is one major cause of anatomical loss of muscle tissue and functional impairment. However, recent data suggest that even bona fide satellite cells (i.e., resident underneath the basal lamina) may be heterogeneous and contain a subpopulation of cells that do not express typical markers such as CD34, Myf5, or M-cadherin and thus represent higher progenitors (Beauchamp et al. 2000).

Dystrophic muscle is also infiltrated by inflammatory cells, mainly lymphocytes and macrophages, followed by fibroblasts that deposit large amounts of collagen contributing to progressive sclerosis of the muscle and adipocytes that also replace muscle with fat tissue. The local microcirculation is progressively lost in this process, leading to a hypoxic condition for surviving or regenerated fibers that activates a vicious circle, increasing the chance of further degeneration.

A series of studies, which followed the original observation of muscle regeneration by bone-marrow-derived cells, demonstrated that additional types of progenitor cells are present in muscle and suggested, although not conclusively, a lineage relationship with bone marrow and resident satellite cells. Work by the Huard group led to the identification of a separate population of late-adhering myogenic cells with several features of self-renewing stem cells. These cells are particularly efficient in restoring a large number of dystrophin positive fibers when injected into mdx muscles (Qu-Petersen et al. 2002). Recent work from the Rudnicki group has shown that in skeletal muscle the SP population is Sca-1 and CD45 positive and can give rise to hematopoietic colonies but not to differentiated muscle unless cocultured with myoblasts or injected into regenerating muscle. This population is different from resident satellite cells that are fractionated as MP (main population), do not express Sca-1 or CD45, and do not form hematopoietic colonies, while expressing myogenic markers and spontaneously differentiating into skeletal muscle. Interestingly, several genetically labeled SP cells could also be found as satellite cells (i.e., underneath the basal lamina and positive for c-Met and M-cadherin) after injection into regenerating muscle, strongly suggesting that at least a fraction of resident satellite cells may have derived from another cell type with SP features (Asakura et al. 2002). Further work by La Barge and Blau (LaBarge and Blau 2002) supported the notion that bone marrow stem cells are at least one source of muscle stem cells and give rise to satellite cells in addition to undergoing immediate muscle differentiation. In the course of this progression, blood-born, bone-marrow-derived cells may respond to local and perhaps systemic signals and cross the vessel layers using a mechanism analogous to leukocytes, to localize initially in a perivascular interstitial district (Tamaki et al. 2002), from which they may be directly recruited to a muscle-forming population or replenish the pool of satellite cells. Acquiring a myogenic identity should imply simultaneous loss of hematopoietic potency. In addition, only hematopoietic stem cells present in skeletal muscle are endowed with the ability to reconstitute lethally irradiated bone marrow (McKinney-Freeman et al. 2002). Surprisingly, a recent report by the Huard group demonstrates that muscle stem cells can differentiate into hematopoietic lineages but retain myogenic potential (Cao et al. 2003). Clearly, the issue still needs to be solved. Similarly to hematopoietic cells, other incoming cells, possibly EPC, may also be incorporated into the endothelium of growing vessels that accompany muscle regeneration and eventually contribute to muscle regeneration. The existence of endothelial-myogenic progenitors in adult muscle (Tamaki et al. 2002) supports this possibility. Since this process probably occurs continuously during life it is possible that any resident satellite cell may derive from the somite-derived myogenic population during embryogenesis or, as we hypothesized before, from incoming cells that may have followed a circulatory route or may have reached developing muscle with the incoming vasculature during fetal angiogenesis. If the latter is the case and these progenitors have a major role in tissue histogenesis, they may play only a minor role in adult tissue homeostasis, being just a remnant of fetal life that is progressively lost after birth. This would explain the low numbers of differentiated muscle cells derived from bone marrow or other tissue and the previous failure of bone marrow transplantation in the mouse model. On the other hand, the case of "mesoangioblasts" that, after in vitro expansion and genetic correction, can be delivered in large numbers to microvasculature of dystrophic muscle, strongly suggest that this route may lead to a successful cell therapy, by exploiting different features of different stem cells to our advantage.

1.7 Future Perspectives

To be successful, a future cell therapy for muscular dystrophy should probably utilize stem cells either derived from the patient (autologous) or from a healthy, immunocompatible donor. In the first case, cells should meet as many as possible of the following criteria: (a) accessible source (e.g., blood, bone marrow, fat aspirate, muscle or skin biopsy), (b) ability to be separated from a heterogeneous population on the basis of antigen expression, (c) potential to grow in vitro for extended periods without loss of differentiation (since it appears currently unlikely that cells may be acutely isolated in numbers sufficient for therapeutic purposes), (d) susceptibility to in vitro transduction with vectors encoding therapeutic genes (these vectors should themselves meet criteria of efficiency, safety, and long term expression), (e) ability to reach the sites of muscle degeneration/regeneration through a systemic route and in response to cytokines released by dystrophic muscle, (f) ability to differentiate in situ into new muscle fibers with high efficiency and to give rise to physiologically normal muscle cells, (g) to be ignored by the immune system, despite the presence of a new protein (the product of the therapeutic gene) and possibly of some residual antigen from the viral vector.

In the case of donor stem cells from an immunocompatible donor, some of the criteria would be less stringent and others more rigorous. For example, the source of the cells would not need to be easily accessible since cells from aborted fetal material may be obtained, including from sites such as the central nervous system, which are not easily accessible in a patient. Gene transduction would not be necessary since donor stem cells would possess a normal copy of the mutated gene. On the other hand, immune suppression would become a major issue in preventing rejection of a classic allograft. While the large amount of experience accumulated in bone marrow transplantation may be essential to devising appropriate protocols, it should also be remembered that some stem cells, for example, mesoangioblasts, do not express class II MHC, making the control of the immune response less complex than in the case of HSC transplantation.

Either way, we are not yet close to meeting all of the required criteria; however, in the last few years (see for example, Cossu and Mavilio 2000) considerable progress has been made in the identification and initial characterization of novel classes of stem cells, some of which have been shown to be able to form skeletal muscle. Furthermore, a replenishment of skeletal muscle myogenic cells by nonresident stem cells has been convincingly demonstrated. Finally, in a mouse model of muscular dystrophy, significant morphological, biochemical, and functional rescue has been achieved by intra-arterial delivery of stem cells. However, functional correction of a large muscle may represent a completely different problem, probably calling for experimentation in a large animal model such as the dystrophic dog. Despite the elevated cost, the need to produce a number of species-specific reagents, the high variability among different dystrophic pups, and the ethical concerns related to the use of dogs for research, it is likely that cell therapy protocols in this animal will bring further information as to the feasibility of similar protocols in dystrophic patients. Hopefully, in a few years time, phase I clinical trials with stem cells may start (Daley 2002) and set the stage for one more, and at least in part successful attack to defeat these genetic diseases.

Acknowledgements. This work was supported by grants from Telethon/Fondazione Zegna, the European Community, Duchenne Parent Project Italia/Compagnia di San Paolo, Muscular Dystrophy Association (USA), Fondazione Istituto Pasteur-Cenci Bolognetti, Associazione Italiana Ricerca sul Cancro (AIRC), Agenzia Spaziale Italiana (ASI) and the Italian Ministry of Health.

References

Asahara T, Murohara T, Sullivan A, Silver M, van der Zee R, Li T, Witzenbichler B, Schatteman G, Isner JM (1997) Isolation of putative progenitor endothelial cells for angiogenesis. Science 275:964–967

Asahara T, Masuda H, Takahashi T, Kalka C, Pastore C, Silver M, Kearne M, Magner M, Isner JM (1999) Bone marrow origin of endothelial progenitor cells responsible for postnatal vasculogenesis in physiological and pathological neovascularization. Circ Res 85:221–228

Asakura A, Seale P, Girgis-Gabardo A, Rudnicki MA (2002) Myogenic specification of side population cells in skeletal muscle. J Cell Biol 159:123–134

Beauchamp JR, Morgan JE, Pagel CN, Partridge TA (1999) Dynamics of myoblast transplantation reveal a discrete minority of precursors with stem cell-like properties as the myogenic source. J Cell Biol 144:1113–1121

Beauchamp JR, Heslop L, Yu DS, Tajbakhsh S, Kelly RG, Wernig A, Buckingham ME, Partridge TA, Zammit PS (2000) Expression of CD34 and Myf5 defines the majority of quiescent adult skeletal muscle satellite cells. J Cell Biol 151:1221–1234

Berghella L, De Angelis L, Coletta M, Berarducci B, Sonnino C, Salvatori G, Anthonissen C, Cooper R, Butler-Browne GS, Mouly V, Ferrari G, Mavilio F, Cossu G (1999) Reversible immortalization of human myogenic cells by site-specific excision of a retrovirally-transferred oncogene. Hum Gene Ther 10:1607–1618

Bianco P, Cossu G (1999) Uno nessuno e centomila. Searching for the identity of mesodermal progenitors. Exptl Cell Res 251:257–263

Bischoff R (1994) The satellite cell and muscle regeneration. In: Engel AG, Franzini-Armstrong C (eds) Myology, 2nd edn. McGraw-Hill, New York, pp 97–133

Blake DJ, Weir A, Newey SE, Davies KE (2002) Function and genetics of dystrophin and dystrophin-related proteins in muscle. Physiol Rev 82:291–329

Burton EA, Davies KE (2002) Muscular dystrophy – reason for optimism? Cell 108:5–8

Cao B, Zheng B, Jankowski RJ, Kimura S, Ikezawa M, Deasy B, Cummins J, Epperly M, Qu-Petersen Z, Huard J (2003) Muscle stem cells differentiate into hematopoietic lineages but retain myogenic potential. Nat Cell Biol (in press)

Cossu G, Clemens P (2001) Gene and cell therapy for muscular dystrophies. In: Emery AH (ed) Muscular dystrophy. Oxford University Press, Oxford, pp 261–283

Cossu G, Mavilio F (2000) Myogenic stem cells for the therapy of primary myopathies: wishful thinking or therapeutic perspective? J Clin Invest 105:1669–1674

Daley GQ (2002) Prospects for stem cell therapeutics: myths and medicines. Curr Opin Genet Dev 12:607–613

De Angelis L, Berghella L, Coletta M, Gabriella Cusella De Angelis M, Lattanzi L, Ponzetto C, Cossu G (1999) Skeletal myogenic progenitors originating from embryonic dorsal aorta co-express endothelial and myogenic markers and contribute to postnatal muscle growth and regeneration. J Cell Biol 147:869–878

De Angelis FG, Sthandier O, Berarducci B, Toso S, Galluzzi G, Ricci E, Cossu G, Bozzoni I (2002) Chimeric snRNA molecules carrying antisense sequences against the splice junctions of exon 51 of the dystrophin pre-mRNA induce exon skipping and restoration of a dystrophin synthesis in Delta 48–50 DMD cells. Proc Natl Acad Sci 99:9456–9461

De Bari C, Dell'Accio F, Vandenabeele F, Vermeesch JR, Raymackers JM, Luyten FP (2003) Skeletal muscle repair by adult human mesenchymal stem cells from synovial membrane. J Cell Biol 160:909–918

Decary S, Mouly V, Hamida CB, Sautet A, Barbet JP, Butler-Browne GS (1997) Replicative potential and telomere length in human skeletal muscle: implications for myogenic cell-mediated gene therapy. Hum Gene Ther 8:1429–1438

Deconinck N, Tinsley J, De Backer F, Fisher R, Kahn D, Phelps S, Davies K, Gillis JM (1997) Expression of truncated utrophin leads to major functional improvements in dystrophen-deficient muscles of mice. Nat Med 3:1216–1221

Duclos F, Straub V, Moore SA, Venzke DP, Hrstka RF, Crosbie RH, Durbeej M, Lebakken CS, Ettinger AJ, van der Meulen J, Holt KH, Lim LE, Sanes JR, Davidson BL, Faulkner JA, Williamson R, Campbell KP (1998) Progressive muscular dystrophy in alpha-sarcoglycan-deficient mice. J Cell Biol 142:1461–1471

Emery AE (2002) The muscular dystrophies. Lancet 317:991–995

Ferrari G, Mavilio F (2002) Myogenic stem cells from the bone marrow: a therapeutic alternative for muscular dystrophy? Neuromuscul Disord 12:S7–S10

Ferrari G, Cusella De Angelis MG, Coletta M, Stornaioulo A, Paolucci E, Cossu G, Mavilio F (1998) Skeletal muscle regeneration by bone marrow derived myogenic progenitors. Science 279:1528–1530

Ferrari G, Stornaioulo A, Mavilio F (2001) Failure to correct murine muscular dystrophy. Nature 411:1014–1015

Friedenstein AJ, Piatetzky S II, Petrakova KV (1966) Osteogenesis in transplants of bone marrow cells. J Embryol Exp Morphol 16(3):381–390

Galli R, Borello U, Gritti A, Giulia Minasi MG, Bjornson C, Coletta M, Mora M, Cusella De Angelis MG, Fiocco R, Cossu G, Vescovi AL (2000) Skeletal myogenic potential of adult neural stem cells. Nat Neurosci 3:986–991

Goodell MA, Brose K, Paradis G, Conner AS, Mulligan RC (1996) Isolation and functional properties of murine hematopoietic stem cells that are replicating in vivo. J Exp Med 183:1797–1806

Grounds MD (1999) Muscle regeneration: molecular aspects and therapeutic implications. Curr Opin Neurol 12:535–543

Guerette BD, Skuk F, Celestin JC, Huard F, Tardif I, Asselin B, Roy M, Goulet R, Roy R, Entman M, Tremblay JP (1997) Prevention by anti-LFA-1 of acute myoblast death following transplantation. J Immunol 159:2522–2531

Gussoni E, Blau HM, Kunkel LM (1997) The fate of individual myoblasts after transplantation into muscles of DMD patients. Nat Med 3:970–977

Gussoni E, Soneoka Y, Strickland CD, Buzney EA, Khan MK, Flint AF, Kunkel LM, Mulligan RC (1999) Dystrophin expression in the mdx mouse restored by stem cell transplantation. Nature 401:390–394

Gussoni E, Bennett RR, Muskiewicz KR, Meyerrose T, Nolta JA, Gilgoff I, Stein J, Chan Y, Lidov HG, Bönnemann CG, von Moers A, Morris GE, den Dunnen JT, Chamberlain JS, Kunkel LM, Weinberg K (2002) Long-term persistence of donor nuclei in a Duchenne muscular dystrophy patient receiving bone marrow transplantation. J Clin Invest 110:807–814

Harper SQ, Hauser MA, DelloRusso C, Duan D, Crawford RW, Phelps ST, Harper HA, Robinson AS, Engelhardt JF, Brooks SV, Chamberlain JS (2002) Modular flexibility of dystrophin: implications for gene therapy of Duchenne muscular dystrophy. Nat Med 8:253–261

Jiang Y, Vaessen B, Lenvik T, Blackstad M, Reyes M, Verfaillie CM (2002a) Multipotent progenitor cells can be isolated from postnatal murine bone marrow, muscle, and brain. Exp Hematol 30:896–904

Jiang Y, Jahagirdar BN, Reinhardt RL, Schwartz RE, Keene CD, Ortiz-Gonzalez XR, Reyes M, Lenvik T, Lund T, Blackstad M, Du J, Aldrich S, Lisberg A, Low WC, Largaespada DA, Verfaillie CM (2002b) Pluripotency of mesenchymal stem cells derived from adult marrow. Nature 418:41–49

Kardon G, Campbell JK, Tabin CJ (2002) Local extrinsic signals determine muscle and endothelial cell fate and patterning in the vertebrate limb. Dev Cell 3:533–545

Kelly R, Alonso S, Tajbakhsh S, Cossu G, Buckingham M (1995) Myosin light chain 3f regulatory sequences confer regionalized cardiac and skeletal muscle expression in transgenic mice. J Cell Biol 129:383–396

Kinoshita I, Roy R, Dugre FJ, Gravel C, Goulet M, Asselin I, Tremblay JP (1996) Myoblast transplantation in monkeys: control of immune response by FK506. J Neuropathol Exp Neurol 55:687–697

Kinoshita I, Vilquin LT, Guerette B, Asselin I, Roy R, Tremblay JP (1994) Very efficient myoblast allotransplantation in mice under Fk-506 immunosuppression. Muscle Nerve 17:1407–1415

LaBarge MA, Blau HM (2002) Biological progression from adult bone marrow to mononucleate muscle stem cell to multinucleate muscle fiber in response to injury. Cell 111:589–601

Lagasse E, Connors H, Al-Dhalimy M, Reitsma M, Dohse M, Osborne L, Wang X, Finegold M, Weissman IL, Grompe M (2000) Purified hematopoietic stem cells can differentiate into hepatocytes in vivo. Nat Med 6:1229–1234

Lattanzi L, Salvatori G, Coletta M, Sonnino C, Cusella De Angelis MG, Gioglio L, Murry CE, Kelly R, Ferrari G, Molinaro M, Crescenzi M, Mavilio F, Cossu G (1998) High efficiency myogenic conversion of human fibroblasts by adenoviral vector-mediated MyoD gene transfer. An alternative strategy for ex vivo gene therapy of primary myopathies. J Clin Invest 101:2119–2128

Liechty KW, Mackenzie TC, Shaaban AF, Radu A, Moseley AB, Deans R, Marshak DR, Flakel AW (2000) Human mesenchymal stem cells engraft and demonstrate site specific differentiation after in utero transplantation in sheep. Nat Med 6:1282–1286

Mauro A (1961) Satellite cell of skeletal muscle fibers. J Biophys Biochem Cytol 9:493–495

McKinney-Freeman SL, Jackson KA, Camargo FD, Ferrari G, Mavilio F, Goodell MA (2002) Muscle-derived hematopoietic stem cells are hematopoietic in origin. Proc Natl Acad Sci 99(3):1341–1346

Minasi MG, Riminucci M, De Angelis L, Borello U, Berarducci B, Innocenzi A, Caprioli A, Sirabella D, Baiocchi M, De Maria R, Jaffredo T, Broccoli V, Bianco P, Cossu G (2002) The meso-angioblast: a multipotent, self-renewing cell that originates from the dorsal aorta and differentiates into most mesodermal tissues. Development 129:2773–2783

Nishino I, Ozawa E (2002) Muscular dystrophies. Curr Opin Neurol 15:539–544

Partridge TA (1996) Myoblast transplantation. In: Lanza RP, Chick WL (eds) Yearbook of cell and tissue transplantation 1996/1997. Kluwer, Netherlands, pp 53–59

Partridge TA, Beauchamp JR, Morgan JE (1989) Conversion of mdx myofibres from dystrophen-negative to -positive by injection of normal myoblasts. Nature 337:176–179

Prockop DJ (1997) Marrow stromal cells as stem cells for non-hematopoietic tissues. Science 276:71–74

Qu-Petersen Z, Deasy B, Jankowski R, Ikezawa M, Cummins J, Pruchnic R, Mytinger J, Cao B, Gates B, Wernig A, Huard J (2002) Identification of a novel population of muscle stem cells in mice: potential for muscle regeneration. J Cell Biol 157:851–864

Reyes M, Lund T, Lenvik T, Aguiar D, Koodie L, Verfaillie CM (2001) Purification and ex vivo expansion of postnatal human marrow mesodermal progenitor cells. Blood 98:2615–2625

Sampaolesi M, Torrente Y, Innocenzi A, Tonlorenzi R, D'Antona G, Pellegrino MA, Barresi R, Bresolin N, Cusella De Angelis MG, Campbell KP, Bottinelli R, Cossu G (2003) Cell therapy of alpha sarcoglycan null dystrophic mice through intra-arterial delivery of mesoangioblasts. Science 301(5632):487–492

Seale P, Asakura A, Rudnicki MA (2001) The potential of muscle stem cells. Dev Cell 1:333–342

Skuka D, Vilquin JT, Tremblay JP (2002) Experimental and therapeutic approaches to muscular dystrophies. Curr Opin Neurol 15:563–569

Tamaki T, Akatsuka A, Ando K, Nakamura Y, Matsuzawa H, Hotta T, Roy RR, Edgerton VR (2002) Identification of myogenic-endothelial progenitor cells in the interstitial spaces of skeletal muscle. J Cell Biol 157:571–577

Torrente Y. Belicchi A, Sampaolesi M, Pisati F, Lestingi M, D'Antona G, Tonlorenzi R, Porretti L, Gavina M, Mamchaoui K, Pellegrino MA, Furling D, Mouly V, Butler-Browne GS, Bottinelli R, Cossu G, Bresolin N (2004) Human circulating AC133+ stem cells replenish the satellite cell pool, resore dystrophin expression and ameliorate function upon transplantation in murine dystrophic skeletal muscle. J Clin Invest (in press)

Wakitani S, Saito T, Caplan AI (1995) Myogenic cells derived from rat bone marrow mesenchymal stem cells exposed to 5-azacytidine. Muscle Nerve 18:1417–1426

Zuk PA, Zhu M, Mizuno H, Huang J, Futrell JW, Katz AJ, Benhaim P, Lorenz HP, Hedrick MH (2001) Multilineage cells from human adipose tissue: implications for cell-based therapies. Tissue Eng 7:211–228

2 Cardiac Myoblasts

P. Menasché

2.1 Introduction

The management of patients with heart failure is receiving a continuously growing interest because of the increased prevalence (approximately 5 million United States citizens) and incidence (400,000–600,000 new patients every year) of this condition. The magnitude of the problem is expected to be even further amplified in the forthcoming years because of the increased age of the population and the improved postinfarction survival rates resulting from recent pharmacological and interventional treatments.

Contemporary medical therapy has dramatically improved the prognosis of heart failure. In many cases, however, medical therapy is simply palliative, and mortality remains high, up to 60% within 1 year for patients in New York Heart Association functional class IV. These figures obviously translate into tremendous financial costs, primarily hospital-driven, which are estimated to consume 1%–2% of the total health care budget of western countries (Berry et al. 2001).

Although cardiac transplantation remains the only radical treatment of the most advanced forms of heart failure, the limitations of this approach, largely related to lack of donor organs and late graft vasculopathy, have led to a continued endeavor for designing alternate options. Most of them have focused on reshaping the dilated left ventricle, primarily by endocardial patch plasty (Dor et al. 1998) and, more recently, by passive constraint devices. In parallel, improvements have been made in ventricular assist devices, particularly as destination therapy (Rose et al. 2001), but the use of permanently implantable blood pumps still remains investigational. In patients with wide QRS complexes, cardiac resynchronization has also emerged as a promising treatment (Young et al. 2003), which does not exclude additional approaches more directly targeted at improving pump function. In this setting, cell transplantation is currently generating a great deal of interest.

2.2 Basic Assumptions

Cell transplantation is based on two major assumptions: (a) heart failure develops when a critical number of cardiomyocytes has been irreversibly lost, and (b) function could thus be improved by repopulating these areas of dysfunctional myocardium with a new pool of contractile cells. Assuming that self-repair endogenous mechanisms, i.e., spontaneous multiplication of adult cardiomyocytes (Kajstura et al. 1998; Beltrami et al. 2001) is too low for compensating for the loss of cardiomyocytes resulting from a large infarct and that conversion of in-scar fibroblasts into contractile cells would require genetic manipulations of questionable clinical relevance, the most realistic approach consists of exogenously supplying a new pool of contractile cells targeted to engraft into the postinfarct scars.

From a conceptual standpoint, the "ideal" cell for transplantation has to meet several stringent criteria: it should be easy to collect and expand, relatively tolerant to ischemia so as to survive in a poorly vascularized scar tissue, and establish connections with host cardiomyocytes allowing its effective and synchronous contribution to heartbeats. Unfortunately, none of the various cell lineages that have been considered so far matches all these requirements.

Quite logically, the initial groundbreaking studies have used fetal and neonatal cardiomyocytes with the reasoning that they would be the most suitable for replacement of lost cardiomyocytes. These experiments have been pivotal to establish "proof-of-concept" in that they have shown, in rodent models of coronary artery ligation or cryoinjury-induced myocardial infarction, that these cells successfully engrafted, were coupled with host cardiomyocytes through connexin 43-supported gap junctions, improved left ventricular function (Leor et al. 1996; Li et al. 1996; Scorsin et al. 1997), and maintained their cardioprotective effects up to 6 months after transplantation (Müller-Ehmsen et al. 2002). However, from a clinical perspective, the transplantation of fetal or neonatal cardiac cells raises significant issues related to ethics, availability, sensitivity to ischemia, the probability of massive graft death, and immunogenicity which question the wide-scale clinical applicability of this approach. Thus, it soon became evident that a way to circumvent these problems was to use stem cells from skeletal muscle, i.e., skeletal myoblasts.

2.3 Skeletal Myoblasts for Cardiac Repair: Experimental Studies

These myogenic precursors (known as satellite cells) normally lie in a quiescent state under the basal membrane of skeletal muscular fibers. Following tissue injury, they are rapidly mobilized, proliferate, and fuse, thereby effecting regeneration of the damaged fibers. In a clinical perspective, these cells feature several attractive characteristics: (a) an autologous origin which overcomes all problems related to availability, ethics, and immunogenicity and is a key factor for large-scale clinical applicability, (b) a high proliferative potential under appropriate culture conditions, (c) a commitment to a well-differentiated myogenic lineage which virtually eliminates the risk of tumorigenicity, and (d) a high resistance to ischemia, which is a major advantage given the hostile environment (postinfarct scars) in which they are to be implanted.

Analysis of the bulk of experimental data on myoblast transplantation, derived from over 45 published papers, was recently reviewed in an editorial comment from one member of the leading group in this area (Minami et al. 2003) and can be summarized as follows. Morphologically, the injected myoblasts differentiate into typical multinucleated myotubes which were shown, in a sheep model of myocardial infarction, to repopulate the areas of fibrosis (Ghostine et al. 2002). Although we and others (Murry et al. 1996) have failed to demonstrate any morphological change of the injected cells into cardiomyocytes, engrafted myotubes coexpress fast, skeletal muscle-type and slow myosin (Murry et al. 1996). Indeed, the proportion of fibers demonstrating a purely slow or composite (fast and slow) myosin isoform pattern increases over time. This observation suggests that factors associated with the myocardial environment (stretch and/or repeated electromechanical stimulation) may lead to some phenotypic adaptation similar to that previously reported after dynamic cardiomyoplasty and this fiber conversion is considered to be potentially beneficial because of the increased resistance of slow-twitch fibers to fatigue and their expected greater ability to withstand a cardiac-type workload. In contrast, however, to fetal cardiomyocytes, engrafted skeletal myotubes do not seem to physically couple with host cardiac cells. Indeed, cultured skeletal myoblasts express N-cadherin and connexin-43 (the major proteins constitutive of fascia adherens and gap junctions and therefore responsible for mechanical and electrical coupling, respectively, in heart tissue) but expression of these proteins is downregulated following intramyocardial implantation (Reinecke et al. 2000). Likewise, our electrophysiological studies show that the membrane properties of engrafted myotubes retain typical skeletal muscle patterns with, for example, action potential durations almost ten times shorter than those of host cardiomyocytes (Léobon et al. 2003).

The functional correlate of these observations is an improvement in left ventricular function, which has been demonstrated in small and large animal models of myocardial infarction created by coronary artery ligation, cryoinjury, or toxic chemicals (Ghostine et al. 2002; Taylor et al. 1998; Kao et al. 2000; Rajnoch et al. 2001; Jain et al. 2001). A causal relationship between the engraftment of cells and the functional outcome is strongly suggested by the data of Taylor et al., who could only document an improved function in cryoin-jured rabbit hearts where autologous myoblasts were successfully identified. Importantly, the functional benefits of myoblast grafting seem to be sustained over time, as suggested by our 1-year follow-up data, which show ejection fraction values unchanged from those measured at the 4-month posttransplant study point (Al Attar et al. 2003). As previously mentioned, this long-term benefit could con-ceivably reflect the fatigue-resistance of the slow-twitch component of the engrafted myotubes. Finally, we (Pouzet et al. 2001) and others (Tambara et al. 2002) have found that the posttransplant im-provement in function was closely related to the number of injected myoblasts (Pouzet et al. 2001), but dose-escalation studies are clearly required to better characterize the relationship between the number of grafted myoblasts and the functional outcome.

The mechanism(s) by which implanted myoblasts improve func-tion have not yet been elucidated and at least three hypotheses, which are not mutually exclusive, can be put forward.

First, the elastic properties of implanted cells could act as a scaf-fold strengthening the ventricular wall and subsequently limiting postinfarct scar expansion. Along this line of reasoning, it is also conceivable that implanted cells secrete factors leading to a reorgani-zation of the extracellular matrix. Thus, one of the remaining ques-tions to be addressed is to determine whether myoblast engraftment is associated with inhibition of matrix metalloproteinases and/or in-crease in the myocardial fibrillar collagen network (Spinale et al. 1999), as an improved structural support for both grafted cells and residual native cardiomyocytes might contribute to limit excessive remodeling. However, although such a mechanism may be operative when cells are injected at a relatively early stage after the infarction, and would thus *prevent* ventricular dilatation, it is less likely that myoblast grafts can *reverse* an already completed remodeling pro-cess, as suggested by our clinical observation of unchanged end dia-stolic volumes in patients having undergone late myoblast implanta-tion in old infarcts.

A second hypothesis is that myoblasts directly contribute to in-crease contractile function. This hypothesis is admittedly challenged by the observation that engrafted myoblasts, although retaining cross-striations suggestive of a persistent functionality, are not physically connected to host cardiomyocytes through connexin 43-supported gap junctions. Furthermore, our electrophysiological studies have failed to show any synchronous beats between skeletal muscle grafts and native cardiomyocytes (Léobon et al. 2003). However, when subjected to strong depolarizing currents, these grafts can give rise to action potentials followed by active contractions, thereby indicating that engrafted myofibers retain their excitable and contractile properties. It is thus conceivable that in areas where grafted and recipient cells are in close physical contact (which may not be uncommon in the human setting where infarcts often feature a patchy pattern), myotubes could be excited by currents fired by the neighboring cardiomyocytes and flowing directly through cell membranes, i.e., bypassing the classical gap junctions pathway. Assuming, however, that this may only occur as a random event, it could be interesting to enhance cell-to-cell communications by engineering myoblasts with the gene encoding connexin 43 (Suzuki et al. 2001).

The third hypothesis is that transplanted cells behave as platforms, releasing growth factors that could mobilize a quiescent pool of cardiac stem cells and consequently trigger an endogenous regeneration. This population has recently been described in the mouse myocardium (Hierlihy et al. 2002) and shown to be recruited and/or activated by factors that attenuate postnatal cardiac growth. Although the phenotypic features of this resident side-population begin to be characterized (it thus appears that these cells are distinct from endothelial or hematopoietic progenitors), many factors remain unknown, including the extent to which activation of these cells can compensate for lost cardiomyocytes and the mediators able to recruit them. In this regard, it is noteworthy that recent data from our laboratory have shown that insulin growth factor-1, a growth factor whose cardioprotective effects have been largely documented (Wang et al. 2001; Welch et al. 2002), was produced by myoblasts and myotubes across a wide variety of species, including human beings. Another study (Behfar et al. 2002) has highlighted the role of a cardiac paracrine transforming growth factor $\beta 1$ and bone morphogenetic protein 2 signaling pathway for driving uncommitted embryonic stem cells towards a cardiomyogenic phenotype. Altogether, these data fit a paradigm whereby engrafted myoblasts would exert beneficial effects on remodeling and/or contractility through the release of mediators acting on endogenous targets. It should be stressed that clarification of the mechanisms by which myoblast transplantation favorably affects function of the infarcted myocardium is not only of cognitive interest but also has practical implications. Namely, if the primary effect of transplantation is to alter remodeling, it should then be performed at a relatively early stage of the disease, within a given time window that needs to be specified. Conversely, if improved function is the result of additional contractile cells replacing the scar area, engraftment should theoretically remain successful at any time point after infarction.

2.4 Skeletal Myoblasts for Cardiac Repair: Clinical Studies

These experimental data have set the stage for three published phase I clinical trials (Siminiak et al. 2002; Dib et al. 2002; Menasché et al. 2003) involving cardiac surgical patients with severe left ventricular dysfunction, postinfarction discrete akinetic and nonviable scars which represent the target for cell injections, and an indication for coronary artery bypass surgery in remote ischemic areas. Skeletal myoblast transplantation has also been performed as a stand-alone procedure using an endoventricular catheter (the results of which have not yet been published). A recent porcine study (chronologically posterior to the human trial) has used iron oxide-loaded myoblasts and magnetic resonance imaging to document the accuracy of these targeted catheter-based implantations into infarcted myocardium (Garot et al. 2003). However, as the assessment was done only 90 min after transplantation, the long-term retention patterns and the differentiation potential of cells injected through an endocardial route still remain to be determined.

Overall, a first lesson gained from these initial studies is that the procedure is quite feasible, i.e., it is possible to grow several hundred million cells from a small muscular biopsy harvested at the thigh. The expansion process extends over 2–3 weeks under Good Manufacturing Practice conditions, and the final cell yield can be concentrated in a small volume (in our experience, 5–6 ml) and surgically injected in multiple sites (approximately 30) across and around the scar without procedural complications. A second important piece of information

pertaining to safety is that myoblast transplantation is potentially proarrhythmic. In our phase I study, four patients out of 10 demonstrated
sustained episodes of ventricular tachycardia and the endoventricular
catheter-based trial had to be temporarily stopped because of two sud-
den deaths presumably due to arrhythmias. This concern, however,
should be tempered by the finding that in patients with a history of
myocardial infarction associated with severe left ventricular dysfunction or congestive heart failure (i.e., patients very similar to those
who comprise the cell transplant population), the risk of postbypass
ventricular tachycardia has been reported to increase up to 30%
(Steinberg et al. 1999). Nevertheless, even if one recognizes that it
is difficult to conclusively establish a causal relationship between ventricular arrhythmias and cell grafting in the absence of control groups
and in a patient population that is in fact prone to develop these types of
events, safety obligations require that this relationship be considered
more than likely until the results of the ongoing randomized trials indicate whether it has to be revisited or not. The mechanism of these
allegedly transplantation-related arrhythmias remains elusive but the
previously mentioned differences in electrical membrane properties between donor and recipient cells could provide a substrate for micro-
reentry circuits. As long as the potential proarrhythmic risk associated
with myoblast transplantation has not been fully elucidated, it has been
deemed safe to recommend implantation of an internal defibrillator, the
legitimacy of which is reinforced by the fact that the characteristics of
this cell transplant patient population tightly overlap those of the MA-
DIT II trial (Moss et al. 2002). Implantation of defibrillators in our
ongoing placebo-controlled randomized trial is of additional cognitive
interest as interrogation of the device will provide a reliable means of
quantifying the incidence of arrhythmias and defining their elective
timing of onset, if any (incidentally, there have been few appropriate
shocks fired by the defibrillators implanted in our phase I patients).

Because of their design (small patient populations, absence of control groups, confounding effect of associated revascularization, lack of
statistical power), these pilot trials do not allow definitive conclusions
pertaining to efficacy. Nevertheless, our findings that approximately
60% of initially akinetic and metabolically nonviable segments recov-
ered some degree of systolic thickening following myoblast implantation (Menasché et al. 2003) are encouraging and consistent with obser-

vations made by the other groups which have evaluated myoblast transplantation. For this reason, we have implemented a large-scale, multicenter randomized study with blinded and centralized contractility of the grafted regions as the primary end point. The additional, although limited, pathological observations made in human hearts (Hagège et al. 2003; Pagani et al. 2003) that myotubes could be detected in the injected areas lend further support to a potential link between engraftment of cells and improvement in function.

2.5 Skeletal Myoblasts for Cardiac Repair:
Future Directions

2.5.1 Comparison with Other Cell Types

Skeletal myoblasts have represented the first generation of cells to be used clinically for the treatment of heart failure, but there is now a great deal of enthusiasm for bone marrow-derived cells. These cells share with myoblasts the possibility of being used as autografts, but they are credited with the additional advantage of an intrinsic plasticity which might allow them to convert to cardiac and/or endothelial cells in response to appropriate culture or environmental conditions. As this issue is addressed in another chapter, the present section will be limited to highlighting the number of as yet unknown factors related to bone marrow-derived cell transplantation (optimal cell subpopulation, method of scale-up, fate of engrafted cells, role of the host-derived signals). It is equally important that the basic studies which try to address these questions include control groups receiving not only culture medium but also skeletal myoblasts, which should now be considered as a benchmark against which other cell types must be tested. A recent study of our laboratory (unpublished data) has thus focused on a face-to-face comparison between human cryopreserved myoblasts and human cryopreserved CD133-positive hematopoietic progenitors in a nude rat model of myocardial infarction. The results document an improved function in the bone marrow-transplanted group compared with controls injected with culture medium alone, but fail to show any superiority of the progenitors over myoblasts. Indeed, our current view is that bone marrow transplantation could be particularly effective for inducing angiogenesis, whereas skeletal myoblasts would be more suitable for myogenesis. Thus, these two cell types might turn out to be more complementary than competitive. Further down the road, embryonic stem cells will also have to be considered as potential cell substitutes for myocardial replacement therapy although they raise major technical, regulatory, and ethical challenges.

2.5.2 Routes of Cell Delivery

So far, cell injections have been mostly accomplished under direct control, through multiple epicardial punctures. To reduce the invasiveness of the procedure, percutaneous approaches are currently undergoing a largely industry-driven extensive development and many of them have already been used in patients despite the scarcity of preclinical data. Theoretically, cells can be injected from the ventricular cavity into the coronary arteries or into the scar tissue through the venous system under electromagnetic, angiographic or echocardiographic guidance. Overall, the experimental evaluation of these various approaches has been limited. One study (Grossman et al. 2002) has reported a higher intramyocardial retention of microspheres after endoventricular injections compared with epicardial injections, a result consistent with the otherwise reported efficacy of transendocardial delivery of bone marrow cells to improve collateral perfusion and function of porcine myocardium. However, the extent to which these data can be extended to myoblasts remains uncertain. As the size of these cells makes hazardous their direct intracoronary injection, whereas endoventricular injections are time-consuming and carry the risk of major cell leakage subsequent to squeezing of the ventricle, we currently favor the transvenous coronary sinus approach, which entails the use of a dedicated catheter featuring an extendable needle along which a microcatheter is advanced and used for staged injections into the postinfarction scar tissue. Efficacy studies are currently ongoing in a sheep model of myocardial infarction and should help to better define the role of this technique among catheter-based approaches.

Regardless of the route of delivery, cell death remains a major limitation of cell transplantation as up to 90% of cells die shortly after injections and it is still unknown to what extent multiplication of those which have survived can catch up this high attrition rate (Zhang et al. 2001). Several factors contribute to cell death, including physical strain during injections, inflammation, apoptosis, and the hypoxic environment inherent in postinfarction scars. Consequently, the development of strategies designed to enhance cell survival is mandatory for optimizing the functional benefits of cell transplantation. Among them, those which are targeted at increasing angiogenesis look particularly promising (Sakakibara et al. 2002).

2.5.3 Extension to Nonischemic Cardiomyopathies

Although most studies have used animal models of ischemic cardiomyopathy, preliminary data now suggest that the benefits of cell transplantation might also extend to globally dilated, idiopathic (Yoo et al. 2000), or drug-induced (Scorsin et al. 1998) cardiomyopathies. Our most recent results with autologous skeletal myoblast transplantation in a Syrian hamster model of dilated cardiomyopathy tend to support these initial findings and, along with the development of percutaneous techniques allowing a widespread cell delivery, might open the way to an extension of indications.

Cell transplantation has now entered the clinical arena and might well find its place in the armamentarium of techniques implemented to improve the outcome of heart failure patients. Nevertheless, several key problems are not fully settled, including the optimal cell type in relation to the objective (i.e., angiogenesis in ischemic patients versus myogenesis in those with heart failure), the means of enhancing cell survival and long-term engraftment, the development of less invasive cell delivery techniques, and the potential applications of cell therapy to nonischemic cardiomyopathies. In the meantime, clinical studies need to more fully assess the safety and efficacy of myoblast (and other cell-based) therapy, but only those designed and powered like drug trials will yield clinically meaningful data. Thus, there is still some time ahead before we know whether the impact of myoblast transplantation on patient outcomes really matches the current expectations.

References

Al Attar N, Carrion C, Ghostine S, Garcin I, Vilquin JT, Hagège AA, Menasché Ph (2003) Long-term (1 year) functional and histological results of autologous skeletal muscle cells transplantation in rat. Cardiovasc Res 58:142–148

Behfar A, Zingman LV, Hodgson DM, et al. (2002) Stem cell differentiation requires a paracrine pathway in the heart. FASEB J 16:1558–1566

Beltrami AP, Urbanek K, Kajstura J, et al. (2001) Evidence that human cardiac myocytes divide after myocardial infarction. N Engl J Med 344:1750–1757

Berry C, Murdoch D, McMurray J (2001) Economics of chronic heart failure. Eur J Heart Failure 3:283–291

Dib N, McCarthy P, Dinsmore J, et al. (2002) Safety and feasibility of autologous myoblast transplantation in patients with ischemic cardiomyopathy: interim analysis from the United States experience (abstract). Circulation 106(II):II-463

Dor V, Sabatier M, Di Donato M, Montiglio F, Toso A, Maioli M (1998) Efficacy of endoventricular patch plasty in large postinfarction akinetic scar and severe left ventricular dysfunction: comparison with a series of large dyskinetic scars. J Thorac Cardiovasc Surg 116:50–59

Fuchs S, Baffour R, Zhou YF, et al. (2001) Transendocardial delivery of autologous bone marrow enhances collateral perfusion and regional function in pigs with chronic experimental myocardial ischemia. J Am Coll Cardiol 37:1726–1732

Garot J, Unterseeh T, Teiger E, et al. (2003) Magnetic resonance imaging of targeted catheter-based implantation of myogenic precursor cells into infarcted left ventricular myocardium. J Am Coll Cardiol 41:1841–1846

Ghostine S, Guarita Sousa LC, Carrion C, et al. (2002) Skeletal myoblast transplantation decreases fibrosis and improves regional function of infarcted myocardial areas. Circulation 106(I):131–136

Grossman PM, Han Z, Palasis M, Barry JJ, Lederman RJ (2002) Incomplete retention after direct myocardial injection. Catheter Cardiovasc Interv 55:392–397

Hagège AA, Carrion C, Menasché Ph, et al. (2003) Autologous skeletal myoblast grafting in ischemic cardiomyopathy. Clinical validation of long-term cell viability and differentiation. Lancet 361:491–492

Hierlihy AM, Seale P, Lobe CG, Rudnicki MA, Megeney LA (2002) The post-natal heart contains a myocardial stem cell population. FEBS Lett 530:239–243

Jain M, DerSimonian H, Brenner DA, et al. (2001) Cell therapy attenuates deleterious ventricular remodeling and improves cardiac performance after myocardial infarction. Circulation 103:1920–1927

Kajstura J, Leri A, Finato N, Di Loreto C, Beltrami CA (1998) Myocyte proliferation in end-stage cardiac failure in humans. Proc Natl Acad Sci 95:8801–8805

Kao RL, Chin TK, Ganote CE, Hossler FE, Li C, Browder W (2000) Satellite cell transplantation to repair injured myocardium. Cardiac Vascular Regeneration 1:31–42

Léobon B, Menasché P, Vilquin JT, Audinat E, Charpak S (2003) Myoblasts transplanted into rat infarcted myocardium are functionally isolated from their host. Proc Natl Acad Sciences 100:7808–7811

Leor J, Patterson M, Quinones MJ, Kedes LH, Kloner RA (1996) Transplantation of fetal myocardial tissue into the infarcted myocardium of rat. Circulation 94 [Suppl II]:332–336

Li R-K, Jia Z-Q, Weisel RD, et al. (1996) Cardiomyocyte transplantation improves heart function. Ann Thorac Surg 62:654–661

Menasché Ph, Hagège AA, Vilquin JT, et al. (2003) Autologous skeletal myoblast transplantation for severe postinfarction left ventricular dysfunction. J Am Coll Cardiol 41:1078–1083

Minami E, Reinecke H, Murry CE (2003) Skeletal muscle meets cardiac muscle. Friends or foes? J Am Coll Cardiol 41:1084–1086

Moss AJ, Zareba W, Hall WJ, et al. (2002) The multicenter automatic defibrillator implantation trial in investigators. Prophylactic implantation of a defibrillator in patients with myocardial infarction and reduced ejection fraction. New Engl J Med 346:877–883

Müller-Ehmsen J, Peterson KL, Kedes L, et al. (2002) Long term survival of transplanted neonatal rat cardiomyocytes after myocardial infarction and effect on cardiac function. Circulation 105:1720–1726

Murry CE, Wiseman RW, Schwartz SM, Hauschka SD (1996) Skeletal myoblast transplantation for repair of myocardial necrosis. J Clin Invest 98: 2512–2523

Pagani F, DerSimonian R, Zawadska A, et al. (2003) Autologous skeletal myoblasts transplanted to ischemia damaged myocardium in humans. J Am Coll Cardiol 41:879–888

Pouzet B, Vilquin J-T, Hagège AA, et al. (2001) Factors affecting functional outcome after autologous skeletal myoblast transplantation. Ann Thorac Surg 71:844–851

Rajnoch C, Chachques J-C, Berrebi A, Bruneval P, Benoit M-O, Carpentier A (2001) Cellular therapy reverses myocardial dysfunction. J Thorac Cardiovasc Surg 121:871–878

Reinecke H, MacDonald GH, Hauschka SD, Murry CE (2000) Electromechanical coupling between skeletal and cardiac muscle: implications for infarct repair. J Cell Biol 149:731–740

Rose EA, Gelijns AC, Moskowitz AJ, et al. (2001) Long-term mechanical left ventricular assistance for endstage heart failure. N Engl J Med 345: 1435–1443

Sakakibara Y, Nishimura K, Tambara K, et al. (2002) Prevascularization with gelatin microspheres containing basic fibroblast growth factor enhances the benefits of cardiomyocyte transplantation. J Thorac Cardiovasc Surg 124:50–56

Scorsin M, Hagège AA, Marotte F, et al. (1997) Does transplantation of cardiomyocytes improve function of infarcted myocardium. Circulation 96 [Suppl II]:188–193

Scorsin M, Hagège AA, Dolizy I, Marotte F, Mirochnik N, Copin H, et al. (1998) Can cellular transplantation improve function in doxorubicin-induced heart failure? Circulation 98 [Suppl II]:151–156

Siminiak T, Kalawski R, Fiszer D, et al. (2002) Transplantation of autologous skeletal myoblasts in the treatment of patients with postinfarction heart failure. Early results of phase I clinical trial (abstract). Circulation 106 [Suppl]:II-626

Spinale FG, Coker ML, Krombach SR, et al. (1999) Matrix metalloproteinase inhibition during the development of congestive heart failure. Circ Res 85:364–376

Steinberg JS, Gaur A, Sciacca R, Tan E (1999) New-onset sustained ventricular tachycardia after cardiac surgery. Circulation 99:903–908

Suzuki K, Brand NJ, Khan MA, et al. (2001) Overexpression of connexin 43 in skeletal myoblasts: relevance to cell transplantation to the heart. J Thoracic Cardiovasc Surg 122:7597–7566

Tambara K, Sakakibara Y, Sakaguchi G, et al. (2002) Transplanted skeletal myoblasts can fully replace the infarcted myocardium when they survive in the host in large numbers (abstract). Circulation 106 [Suppl II]:549

Taylor DA, Atkins BZ, Hungspreugs P, et al. (1998) Regenerating functional myocardium: improved performance after skeletal myoblast transplantation. Nat Med 4:929–933

Wang PH (2001) Roads to survival. Insulin-like growth factor-1 signaling pathways in cardiac muscle. Circ Res 88:552–554

Welch S, Plank D, Witt S, et al. (2002) Cardiac-specific IGF-1 expression attenuates dilated cardiomyopathy in tropomodulin-expressing transgenic mice. Circ Res 90:641–648

Yoo KJ, Li RK, Weisel RD, et al. (2000) Heart cell transplantation improves heart function in dilated cardiomyopathic hamsters. Circulation 102 [Suppl III]:204–209

Young JB, Abraham WT, Smith AL, et al. (2003) Combined cardiac resynchronization and implantable cardioversion defibrillation in advanced chronic heart failure: the MIRACLE ICD Trial. JAMA 289:2685–2694

Zhang M, Methot D, Poppa V, Fujio Y, Walsh K, Murry CE (2001) Cardiomyocyte grafting for cardiac repair: graft cell death and anti-death strategies. J Mol Cell Cardiol 33:907–921

3 Tissue Engineering, Stem Cells, and Cloning: Current Concepts and Future Trends

C. J. Koh, A. Atala

3.1 Introduction

After flying the first solo transatlantic flight, Charles Lindbergh spent the rest of his life working with Alexis Carrell, a Nobel Laureate in medicine, at the Rockefeller Institute in New York culturing organs in the hope of using cells and tissues for future transplantation. Together, Carrell and Lindbergh published a book in 1938, titled "The Culture of Organs" (Carrel and Lindbergh 1938). Organ cultures of many different tissue types were described in their seminal work.

Over 60 years later, the culture and expansion of cells for transplantation and the engineering of various tissues has become routine. Over the last decade, the ability to use cells for therapy and to engineer tissues has broadened the theoretical options for tissue reconstruction and organ transplantation. Nonetheless, the road towards the replacement of tissue and organ function has been arduous. Organ transplantation was not possible until 1954 when Joseph Murray performed the first successful kidney transplant from an identical twin into his brother (Murray et al. 1955). In the early 1960s, Murray performed a nonrelated kidney transplant from a nongenetically identical patient into another. This transplant, which overcame the immunological barrier, marked a new era in medical therapy, where transplantation could be used as a means of therapy for different organ systems. However, the lack of adequate immunosuppression, the limited ability to monitor and control rejection, and a severe organ donor shortage, has opened the door for other alternatives.

As times evolved, synthetic materials were developed in order to replace or rebuild diseased tissues or parts in the human body. The advent of new man-made materials, such as Teflon and Silicone, led to the production of a wide array of devices that could be applied for human use. Although these devices could provide structural replacement, the functional component of the original tissue was not replaced. Meanwhile, an increasing body of knowledge in the biological sciences was rapidly growing, which included new techniques for cell harvesting, culture, and expansion. In particular, the areas of cell biology, molecular biology, and biochemistry were advancing rapidly. Studies of the extracellular matrix and its interaction with cells as well as with growth factors and their ligands, gave way to an improved understanding of cell and tissue growth and differentiation. In the 1960s, a natural evolution occurred wherein researchers started to combine the field of devices and material sciences with cell biology. This has led scientists to attempt to use cells for therapy and for the engineering of virtually every tissue of the human body. More recently, major advances in the areas of stem cell biology, tissue engineering, and nuclear transfer techniques have made it possible to combine these technologies, thus creating a field termed Regenerative Medicine.

The body is exposed to a variety of possible injuries from the time the fetus develops. Aside from congenital abnormalities, individuals may also suffer from acquired disorders such as cancer, trauma, infection, inflammation, iatrogenic injuries, or other conditions which may lead to organ damage or loss, requiring eventual reconstruction. The type of native autologous tissue chosen for replacement depends on which organ requires reconstruction. For example, patients with vaginal cancer may have the neoplastic tissue replaced with skin, small bowel, sigmoid colon, and rectum. However, a shortage of the patient's own tissues may limit these types of reconstructions, and there is a degree of morbidity associated with the harvest procedure. In addition, these approaches rarely replace the entire function of the original organ. The tissues used for reconstruction may lead to complications due to their inherently different functional parameters. In most cases, the replacement of lost or deficient tissues with functionally equivalent tissues would improve the outcome for these patients. This goal may be attainable with the use of regenerative medicine techniques.

3.2 Tissue Engineering Principles

As one of the major components of regenerative medicine, tissue engineering follows the principles of cell transplantation, materials science and engineering towards the development of biological substitutes which can restore and maintain normal function. Tissue engineering strategies generally fall into two categories: acellular matrices, where matrices are used alone and which depend on the body's natural ability to regenerate for proper orientation and direction of new tissue growth, and matrices with cells. Acellular tissue matrices are usually prepared by removing cellular components from tissues via mechanical and chemical manipulation to produce collagen-rich matrices (Chen et al. 1999a; Dahms et al. 1998; Piechota et al. 1998; Yoo et al. 1998b). These matrices tend to slowly degrade on implantation and are generally replaced by the extracellular matrix (ECM) proteins that are secreted by the ingrowing cells.

When cells are used for tissue engineering, a small piece of donor tissue is dissociated into individual cells. These cells are either implanted directly into the host, or are expanded in culture, attached to a support matrix, and then reimplanted into the host after expansion. The source of donor tissue can be heterologous (such as bovine), allogeneic (same species, different individual), or autologous. Ideally, both structural and functional tissue replacement will occur with minimal complications. The most preferred cells to use are autologous cells, where a biopsy of tissue is obtained from the host, the cells are dissociated and expanded in culture, and the expanded cells are implanted into the same host (Amiel and Atala 1999a; Atala et al. 1993b, 1994a, 1999; Atala and Lanza 2001; Atala and Mooney 1997; Cilento et al. 1994; Fauza et al. 1998a, b; Godbey and Atala 2002; Kershen and Atala 1999a; Machluf and Atala 1998; Oberpenning et al. 1999; Park et al. 1999; Yoo and Atala 1997; Yoo et al. 1998a, b, 1999). The use of autologous cells avoids rejection, and thus the deleterious side effects of immunosuppressive medications can be avoided.

One of the limitations of applying cell-based regenerative medicine techniques towards organ replacement has been the inherent difficulty of growing specific cell types in large quantities. Even when some organs, such as the liver, have a high regenerative capacity in vivo, cell growth and expansion in vitro may be difficult. By studying the privileged sites for committed precursor cells in specific organs, as well as exploring the conditions that promote differentiation, one may be able to overcome the obstacles that could lead to cell expansion in vitro. For example, urothelial cells could be grown in the laboratory setting in the past, but only with limited expansion. Several protocols were developed over the last two decades which identified the undifferentiated cells, and kept them undifferentiated during their growth phase (Cilento et al. 1994; Liebert et al. 1997;

Puthenveettil et al. 1999; Scriven et al. 1997). Using these methods of cell culture, it is now possible to expand a urothelial strain from a single specimen which initially covers a surface area of 1 cm^2 to one covering a surface area of 4,202 m^2 (the equivalent area of one football field) within 8 weeks (Cilento et al. 1994). These studies indicated that it should be possible to collect autologous bladder cells from human patients, expand them in culture, and return them to the human donor in sufficient quantities for reconstructive purposes (Cilento et al. 1994; Fauza et al. 1998a; Freeman et al. 1997; Harriss 1995; Liebert et al. 1991, 1997; Lobban et al. 1998; Nguyen et al. 1999; Puthenveettil et al. 1999; Rackley et al. 1999; Solomon et al. 1998; Tobin et al. 1994). Major advances have been achieved within the last decade on the possible expansion of a variety of primary human cells, with specific techniques that make the use of autologous cells possible for clinical application.

3.3 Stem Cells

Most current strategies for tissue engineering depend upon a sample of autologous cells from the diseased organ of the host. However, for many patients with extensive end-stage organ failure, a tissue biopsy may not yield enough normal cells for expansion and transplantation. In other instances, primary autologous human cells can not be expanded from a particular organ, such as the pancreas. In these situations, pluripotent human embryonic stem cells are envisioned as a viable source of cells, as they can serve as an alternative source of cells from which the desired tissue can be derived. Combining the techniques learned in tissue engineering over the past few decades with this potentially endless source of versatile cells could lead to novel sources of replacement organs.

Embryonic stem cells exhibit two remarkable properties: the ability to proliferate in a undifferentiated, but pluripotent state (self-renew), and the ability to differentiate into many specialized cell types (Brivanlou et al. 2003). They can be isolated by immunosurgery from the inner cell mass of the embryo during the blastocyst stage (5 days postfertilization), and are usually grown on feeder layers consisting of mouse embryonic fibroblasts or human feeder cells

(Richards et al. 2002). More recent reports have shown that these cells can be grown without the use of a feeder layer (Amit et al. 2003), and thus avoid the exposure of these human cells to mouse viruses and proteins. These cells have demonstrated longevity in culture by maintaining their undifferentiated state for at least 80 passages when grown using current published protocols (Reubinoff et al. 2000; Thomson et al. 1998).

Human embryonic stem cells have been shown to differentiate into cells from all three embryonic germ layers in vitro. Skin and neurons have been formed, indicating ectodermal differentiation (Reubinoff et al. 2001; Schuldiner et al. 2000, 2001; Zhang et al. 2001). Blood, cardiac cells, cartilage, endothelial cells, and muscle have been formed, indicating mesodermal differentiation (Kaufman et al. 2001; Kehat et al. 2001; Levenberg et al. 2002). And pancreatic cells have been formed, indicating endodermal differentiation (Assady et al. 2001). In addition, as further evidence of their pluripotency, embryonic stem cells can form embryoid bodies, which are cell aggregations that contain all three embryonic germ layers, while in culture, and can form teratomas in vivo (Itskovitz-Eldor et al. 2000).

3.4 Therapeutic Cloning

Nuclear cloning, which has also been called nuclear transplantation and nuclear transfer, involves the introduction of a nucleus from a donor cell into an enucleated oocyte to generate an embryo with a genetic makeup identical to that of the donor.

While there has been tremendous interest in the field of nuclear cloning since the birth of Dolly in 1997, the first successful nuclear transfer was reported over 50 years ago by Briggs and King (Briggs and King 1952). Cloned frogs, which were the first vertebrates derived from nuclear transfer, were subsequently reported by Gurdon in 1962 (Gurdon 1962), but the nuclei were derived from nonadult sources. In the past 6 years, tremendous advances in nuclear cloning technology have been reported, indicating the relative immaturity of the field. Dolly was not the first cloned mammal to be produced from adult cells; in fact, live lambs were produced in 1996 using nuclear transfer and differentiated epithelial cells derived from embryonic discs (Campbell et al. 1996). The significance of Dolly was that she was the first mammal to be derived from an adult somatic cell using nuclear transfer (Wilmut et al. 1997). Since then, animals from several species have been grown using nuclear transfer technology, including cattle (Cibelli et al. 1998), goats (Baguisi et al. 1999; Keefer et al. 2002), mice (Wakayama et al. 1998), and pigs (Betthauser et al. 2000; De Sousa et al. 2002; Onishi et al. 2000; Polejaeva et al. 2000).

Two types of nuclear cloning, reproductive cloning and therapeutic cloning, have been described, and a better understanding of the differences between the two types may help to alleviate some of the controversy that surrounds these revolutionary technologies (Colman and Kind 2000; Vogelstein et al. 2002). Banned in most countries for human applications, reproductive cloning is used to generate an embryo that has the identical genetic material as its cell source. This embryo can then be implanted into the uterus of a female to give rise to an infant that is a clone of the donor. On the other hand, therapeutic cloning is used to generate early stage embryos that are explanted in culture to produce embryonic stem cell lines whose genetic material is identical to that of its source. These autologous stem cells have the potential to become almost any type of cell in the adult body, and thus would be useful in tissue and organ replacement applications (Hochedlinger and Jaenisch 2003). Some useful applications would be in the treatment of diseases, such as end-stage kidney disease, neurodegenerative diseases, and diabetes, for which there is limited availability of immunocompatible tissue transplants.

Therefore, therapeutic cloning, which has also been called somatic cell nuclear transfer, provides an alternative source of transplantable cells that theoretically may be limitless. Figure 1 shows the strategy of combining therapeutic cloning with tissue engineering to develop tissues and organs. According to data from the Centers for Disease Control, it has been estimated that approximately 3,000 Americans die every day of diseases that could have been treated with embryonic stem cell-derived tissues (Lanza et al. 2001). With current allogeneic tissue transplantation protocols, rejection is a frequent complication because of immunologic incompatibility, and immunosuppressive drugs are usually administered to treat and hopefully prevent host-versus-graft disease (Hochedlinger and

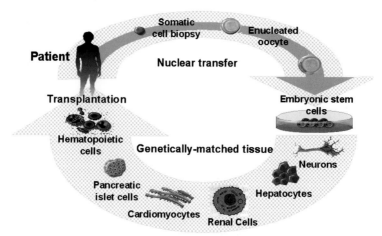

Fig. 1. Strategy for therapeutic cloning and tissue engineering

Jaenisch 2003). The use of transplantable tissue and organs derived from therapeutic cloning may lead to the avoidance of immune responses that typically are associated with transplantation of nonautologous tissues. As a result, with therapeutic cloning, the variety of serious and potentially life-threatening complications associated with immunosuppressive treatments may be avoided (Lanza et al. 1999).

3.5 Biomaterials for Regenerative Medicine

For cell-based tissue engineering, the expanded cells are seeded onto a scaffold synthesized with the appropriate biomaterial. In tissue engineering, biomaterials replicate the biologic and mechanical function of the native extracellular matrix (ECM) found in tissues in the body by serving as an artificial ECM. As a result, biomaterials provide a three-dimensional space for the cells to form into new tissues with appropriate structure and function, and also can allow for the delivery of cells and appropriate bioactive factors (e.g., cell adhesion peptides, growth factors), to desired sites in the body (Kim and Mooney 1998). As the majority of mammalian cell types are anchorage-dependent and will die if no cell-adhesion substrate is available, biomaterials provide a cell-adhesion substrate that can deliver cells to specific sites in the body with high loading efficiency. Biomaterials can also provide mechanical support against in vivo forces such that the predefined three-dimensional structure is maintained during tissue development. Furthermore, bioactive signals, such as cell-adhesion peptides and growth factors, can be loaded along with cells to help regulate cellular function.

The ideal biomaterial should be biocompatible in that it is biodegradable and bioresorbable to support the replacement of normal tissue without inflammation. Incompatible materials are destined for an inflammatory or foreign-body response that eventually leads to rejection and/or necrosis. In addition, the degradation products, if produced, should be removed from the body via metabolic pathways at an adequate rate that keeps the concentration of these degradation products in the tissues at a tolerable level (Bergsma et al. 1995). Furthermore, the biomaterial should provide an environment in which appropriate regulation of cell behavior (e.g., adhesion, proliferation, migration, differentiation) can occur such that functional tissue can form. Cell behavior in the newly formed tissue has been shown to be regulated by multiple interactions of the cells with their microenvironment, including interactions with cell-adhesion ligands (Hynes 1992) and with soluble growth factors (Deuel 1997). In addition, biomaterials provide temporary mechanical support that allows the tissue to grow in three dimensions while the cells undergo spatial tissue reorganization. The properly chosen biomaterial should allow the engineered tissue to maintain sufficient mechanical integrity to support itself in early development, while in late development, the properly-chosen biomaterial should have begun degradation such that it does not hinder further tissue growth (Kim and Mooney 1998).

Generally, three classes of biomaterials have been utilized for engineering tissues: naturally-derived materials (e.g., collagen and alginate), acellular tissue matrices (e.g., bladder submucosa and small intestinal submucosa), and synthetic polymers [e.g., polyglycolic acid (PGA), polylactic acid (PLA), and poly(lactic-co-glycolic acid) (PLGA)]. These classes of biomaterials have been tested with respect to their biocompatibility (Pariente et al. 2001, 2002). Naturally-derived materials and acellular tissue matrices have the potential advantage of biological recognition. However, synthetic polymers can be produced reproducibly on a large scale with controlled properties of their strength, degradation rate, and microstructure.

Collagen is the most abundant and ubiquitous structural protein in the body, and may be readily purified from both animal and human tissues with an enzyme treatment and salt/acid extraction (Li 1995). Collagen implants degrade through a sequential attack by lysosomal enzymes. The in vivo resorption rate can be regulated by controlling the density of the implant and the extent of intermolecular crosslinking. The lower the density, the greater the interstitial space and generally the larger the pores for cell infiltration, leading to a higher rate of implant degradation. Collagen contains cell-adhesion domain sequences (e.g., RGD) which exhibit specific cellular interactions. This may assist to retain the phenotype and activity of many types of cells, including fibroblasts (Silver and Pins 1992) and chondrocytes (Sams and Nixon 1995).

Alginate, a polysaccharide isolated from sea weed, has been used as an injectable cell delivery vehicle (Smidsrod and Skjak-Braek 1990) and a cell immobilization matrix (Lim and Sun 1980) owing to its gentle gelling properties in the presence of divalent ions such as calcium. Alginate is relatively biocompatible and approved by the FDA for human use as wound dressing material. Alginate is a family of copolymers of D-mannuronate and L-guluronate. The physical and mechanical properties of alginate gel are strongly correlated with the proportion and length of polyguluronate block in the alginate chains (Smidsrod and Skjak-Braek 1990).

Acellular tissue matrices are collagen-rich matrices prepared by removing cellular components from tissues. The matrices are often prepared by mechanical and chemical manipulation of a segment of tissue (Chen et al. 1999b; Dahms et al. 1998; Piechota et al. 1998; Yoo et al. 1998c). The matrices slowly degrade upon implantation, and are replaced and remodeled by ECM proteins synthesized and secreted by transplanted or ingrowing cells.

Polyesters of naturally occurring α-hydroxy acids, including PGA, PLA, and PLGA, are widely used in tissue engineering. These polymers have gained FDA approval for human use in a variety of applications, including sutures (Gilding 1981). The ester bonds in these polymers are hydrolytically labile, and these polymers degrade by nonenzymatic hydrolysis. The degradation products of PGA, PLA, and

PLGA are nontoxic, natural metabolites and are eventually eliminated from the body in the form of carbon dioxide and water (Gilding 1981). The degradation rate of these polymers can be tailored from several weeks to several years by altering crystallinity, initial molecular weight, and the copolymer ratio of lactic to glycolic acid. Since these polymers are thermoplastics, they can be easily formed into a three-dimensional scaffold with a desired microstructure, gross shape and dimension by various techniques, including molding, extrusion (Freed et al. 1994), solvent casting (Mikos et al. 1994), phase separation techniques, and gas foaming techniques (Harris et al. 1998). Many applications in tissue engineering often require a scaffold with high porosity and ratio of surface area to volume. Other biodegradable synthetic polymers, including poly(anhydrides) and poly(ortho-esters), can also be used to fabricate scaffolds for tissue engineering with controlled properties (Peppas and Langer 1994).

3.6 Tissue Engineering of Specific Structures

Investigators around the world, including our laboratory, have been working towards the development of several cell types and tissues and organs for clinical application.

3.6.1 Urethra

Various biomaterials without cells, such as PGA and acellular collagen-based matrices from small intestine and bladder, have been used experimentally (in animal models) for the regeneration of urethral tissue (Atala et al. 1992; Bazeed et al. 1983; Chen et al. 1999a; Kropp et al. 1998; Olsen et al. 1992; Sievert et al. 2000). Some of these biomaterials, like acellular collagen matrices derived from bladder submucosa, have also been seeded with autologous cells for urethral reconstruction. Our laboratory has been able to replace tubularized urethral segments with cell-seeded collagen matrices.

Acellular collagen matrices derived from bladder submucosa by our laboratory have been used experimentally and clinically. In animal studies, segments of the urethra were resected and replaced with

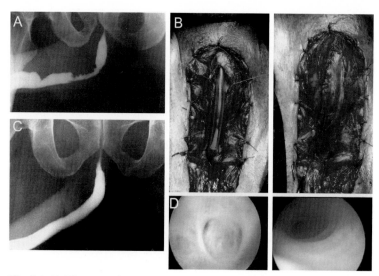

Fig. 2 A–D. Tissue engineering of the urethra using a collagen matrix. **A** Representative case of a patient with a bulbar stricture. **B** Urethral repair. Strictured tissue is excised, preserving the urethral plate on the *left* side, and matrix is anastomosed to the urethral plate in an onlay fashion on the *right*. **C** Urethrogram 6 months after repair. **D** Cystoscopic view of urethra before surgery on the *left* side and 4 months after repair on the *right* side

acellular matrix grafts in an onlay fashion. Histological examination showed complete epithelialization and progressive vessel and muscle infiltration, and the animals were able to void through the neourethras (Chen et al. 1999a). These results were confirmed in a clinical study of patients with hypospadias and urethral stricture disease (El-Kassaby et al. 2003; Yoo et al. 1999). Decellularized cadaveric bladder submucosa was used as an onlay matrix for urethral repair in patients with stricture disease and hypospadias (Fig. 2). Patent, functional neo-urethras were noted in these patients with up to a 7-year follow-up. The use of an off-the-shelf matrix appears to be beneficial for patients with abnormal urethral conditions, and obviates the need for obtaining autologous grafts, thus decreasing operative time and eliminating donor site morbidity.

Unfortunately, the above techniques are not applicable for tubularized urethral repairs. The collagen matrices are able to replace ure-

thral segments only when used in an onlay fashion. However, if a tubularized repair is needed, the collagen matrices should be seeded
with autologous cells to avoid the risk of stricture formation and
poor tissue development (De Filippo et al. 2002a, b). Therefore, tubularized collagen matrices seeded with autologous cells can be
used successfully for total penile urethra replacement.

3.6.2 Bladder

Currently, gastrointestinal segments are commonly used as tissues for
bladder replacement or repair. However, gastrointestinal tissues are designed to absorb specific solutes, whereas bladder tissue is designed for
the excretion of solutes. Due to the problems encountered with the use
of gastrointestinal segments, numerous investigators have attempted
alternative materials and tissues for bladder replacement or repair.

The success of using cell transplantation strategies for bladder reconstruction depends on the ability to use donor tissue efficiently
and to provide the right conditions for long term survival, differentiation, and growth. Urothelial and muscle cells can be expanded in
vitro, seeded onto polymer scaffolds, and allowed to attach and form
sheets of cells (Atala et al. 1993b). These principles were applied
toward the creation of tissue engineered bladders in an animal model that required a subtotal cystectomy with subsequent replacement
with a tissue-engineered organ in beagle dogs (Oberpenning et al.
1999). Urothelial and muscle cells were separately expanded from
an autologous bladder biopsy, and seeded onto a bladder-shaped biodegradable polymer scaffold. The results from this study showed
that it is possible to tissue engineer bladders, which are anatomically
and functionally normal. Clinical trials for the application of this
technology are currently being conducted.

3.6.3 Male Genital Tissues

Reconstructive surgery is required for a wide variety of pathologic
penile conditions, such as penile carcinoma, trauma, severe erectile
dysfunction and congenital conditions like ambiguous genitalia, hy-

pospadias, and epispadias. One of the major limitations of phallic reconstructive surgery is the scarcity of sufficient autologous tissue. Phallic reconstruction using autologous tissue, derived from the patient's own cells, may be preferable in selected cases.

The major components of the phallus are corporal smooth muscle and endothelial cells. The creation of autologous functional and structural corporal tissue de novo would be beneficial. Autologous cavernosal smooth muscle and endothelial cells were harvested, expanded, and seeded on acellular collagen matrices and implanted in a rabbit model (Kershen et al. 2002; Kwon et al. 2002). Histologic examination confirmed the appropriate organization of penile tissue phenotypes, and structural and functional studies, including cavernosography, cavernosometry, and mating studies, demonstrated that it is possible to engineer autologous functional penile tissue. Our laboratory is currently working on increasing the size of the engineered constructs.

3.6.4 Female Genital Tissues

Congenital malformations of the uterus may have profound implications clinically. Patients with cloacal exstrophy and intersex disorders may not have sufficient uterine tissue present for future reproduction. We investigated the possibility of engineering functional uterine tissue using autologous cells (Wang et al. 2003). Autologous rabbit uterine smooth muscle and epithelial cells were harvested, then grown and expanded in culture. These cells were seeded onto preconfigured uterine-shaped biodegradable polymer scaffolds, which were then used for subtotal uterine tissue replacement in the corresponding autologous animals. Upon retrieval 6 months after implantation, histological, immunocytochemical, and Western blot analyses confirmed the presence of normal uterine tissue components. Biomechanical analyses and organ bath studies showed that the functional characteristics of these tissues were similar to those of normal uterine tissue. Breeding studies using these engineered uteri are currently being performed.

Similarly, several pathologic conditions, including congenital malformations and malignancy, can adversely affect normal vaginal development or anatomy. Vaginal reconstruction has traditionally been challenging due to the paucity of available native tissue. The feasibility of engineering vaginal tissue in vivo was investigated (De Filippo et al. 2003 b). Vaginal epithelial and smooth muscle cells of female rabbits were harvested, grown, and expanded in culture. These cells were seeded onto biodegradable polymer scaffolds, and the cell-seeded constructs were then implanted into nude mice for up to 6 weeks. Immunocytochemical, histological, and Western blot analyses confirmed the presence of vaginal tissue phenotypes. Electrical field stimulation studies in the tissue-engineered constructs showed similar functional properties to those of normal vaginal tissue. When these constructs were used for autologous total vaginal replacement, patent vaginal structures were noted in the tissue-engineered specimens, while the noncell-seeded structures were noted to be stenotic (De Filippo et al. 2003 a).

3.6.5 Kidney and Muscle

We applied the principles of both tissue engineering and therapeutic cloning in an effort to produce genetically identical renal, cardiac, and skeletal muscle tissue in a large animal model, the cow (*Bos taurus*; Lanza et al. 2002). Bovine skin fibroblasts from adult Holstein steers were obtained by ear notch, and single donor cells were isolated and microinjected into the perivitelline space of donor enucleated oocytes (nuclear transfer). The resulting blastocysts were implanted into progestrin-synchronized recipients to allow for further in vivo growth. After 12 weeks, cloned renal and muscle cells were harvested, expanded in vitro, then seeded onto biodegradable scaffolds. The constructs, which consisted of the cells and the scaffolds, were then implanted into the subcutaneous space of the same steer from which the cells were cloned to allow for tissue growth.

Histologic examination of the cloned muscle constructs revealed well-organized cellular organization with spindle-shaped nuclei (Fig. 3 A), and immunohistochemical analysis identified muscle fibers within the implanted constructs. In addition, semiquantitative RT-PCR and Western blot analysis confirmed the expression of muscle-specific mRNA and proteins. Furthermore, histologic examination revealed extensive vascularization within the implants, which is essential for the survival and future growth of the cloned tissue.

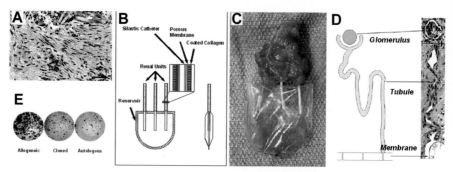

Fig. 3 A–E. Combining therapeutic cloning and tissue engineering to produce kidney and muscle tissue. **A** Retrieved cloned cardiac muscle tissue shows a well-organized cellular orientation 6 weeks after implantation. **B** Illustration of the tissue-engineered renal unit. **C** Renal unit seeded with cloned cells, 3 months after implantation, showing the accumulation of urine-like fluid. **D** There was a clear unidirectional continuity between the mature glomeruli, their tubules, and the polycarbonate membrane. **E** Elispot analyses of the frequencies of T cells that secrete IFN-gamma after primary and secondary stimulation with allogeneic renal cells, cloned renal cells, or nuclear donor fibroblasts

The kidney is a complex organ with multiple cell types and a complex functional anatomy that renders it one of the most difficult to reconstruct (Amiel and Atala 1999 b; Auchincloss and Bonventre 2002). Previous efforts in tissue engineering of the kidney have been directed toward the development of extracorporeal renal support systems made of biological and synthetic components (Aebischer et al. 1987; Amiel et al. 2000; Humes et al. 1999; Ip et al. 1988; Joki et al. 2001; Lanza et al. 1996; MacKay et al. 1998), and ex vivo renal replacement devices are known to be life-sustaining. However, there would be obvious benefits for patients with end-stage kidney disease if these devices could be implanted long-term without the need for an extracorporeal perfusion circuit or immunosuppressive drugs.

Cloned renal cells were seeded on scaffolds consisting of three collagen-coated cylindrical polycarbonate membranes (Fig. 3 B). The ends of the three membranes of each scaffold were connected to catheters that terminated into a collecting reservoir. This created a renal neo-organ with a mechanism for collecting the excreted urinary fluid (Fig. 3 C). These scaffolds with the collecting devices were transplanted subcutaneously into the same steer from which the genetic material originated, and then retrieved 12 weeks after implantation.

Chemical analysis of the collected urine-like fluid, including urea nitrogen and creatinine levels, electrolyte levels, specific gravity, and glucose concentration, revealed that the implanted renal cells possessed filtration, reabsorption, and secretory capabilities.

Histologic examination of the retrieved implants revealed extensive vascularization and self-organization of the cells into glomeruli- and tubule-like structures. A clear continuity between the glomeruli, the tubules, and the polycarbonate membrane was noted that allowed the passage of urine into the collecting reservoir (Fig. 3D). Immunohistochemical analysis with renal-specific antibodies revealed the presence of renal proteins; RT-PCR analysis confirmed the transcription of renal specific RNA in the cloned specimens, and Western blot analysis confirmed the presence of elevated renal-specific protein levels.

Since previous studies have shown that bovine clones harbor the oocyte mitochondrial DNA (Evans et al. 1999; Hiendleder et al. 1999; Steinborn et al. 2000), the donor egg's mitochondrial DNA was thought to be a potential source of immunologic incompatibility. Differences in mtDNA-encoded proteins expressed by cloned cells could stimulate a T-cell response specific for mt-DNA-encoded minor histocompatibility antigens when the cloned cells are implanted back into the original nuclear donor (Fischer Lindahl et al. 1991). We used nucleotide sequencing of the mtDNA genomes of the clone and fibroblast nuclear donor to identify potential antigens in the muscle constructs. Only two amino acid substitutions were noted to distinguish the clone and the nuclear donor, and as a result, a maximum of two minor histocompatibility antigens could be defined. Given the lack of knowledge regarding peptide-binding motifs for bovine MHC class I molecules, there is no reliable method to predict the impact of these amino acid substitutions on bovine histocompatibility.

Oocyte-derived mtDNA was also thought to be a potential source of immunologic incompatibility in the cloned renal cells. Maternally transmitted minor histocompatibility antigens in mice have been shown to stimulate both skin allograft rejection in vivo and cytotoxic T lymphocytes expansion in vitro (Fischer Lindahl et al. 1991) that could prevent the use of these cloned constructs in patients with chronic rejection of major histocompatibility matched human renal transplants (Hadley et al. 1992; Yard et al. 1993). We tested for a possible T-cell response to the cloned renal devices using delayed-type hypersensitivity testing in vivo and Elispot analysis of interferon-gamma secreting T-cells in vitro. Both analyses revealed that the cloned renal cells showed no evidence of a T-cell response, suggesting that rejection will not necessarily occur in the presence of oocyte-derived mitochondrial DNA (Fig. 3E). This finding may represent a step forward in overcoming the histocompatibility problem of stem cell therapy (Auchincloss and Bonventre 2002).

These studies demonstrated that cells derived from nuclear transfer can be successfully harvested, expanded in culture, and transplanted in vivo with the use of biodegradable scaffolds on which the single suspended cells can organize into tissue structures that are genetically identical to that of the host. These studies were the first demonstration of the use of therapeutic cloning for regeneration of tissues in vivo.

3.6.6 Blood Vessels

Xenogenic or synthetic materials have been used as replacement blood vessels for complex cardiovascular lesions. However, these materials typically lack growth potential, and may place the recipient at risk for complications such as stenosis, thromboembolization, or infection (Matsumura et al. 2003).

Tissue-engineered vascular grafts have been constructed using autologous cells and biodegradable scaffolds and have been applied in dog and lamb models (Shinoka et al. 1995, 1996, 1997, 1998; Watanabe et al. 2001). The key advantage from using these autografts is that they degrade in vivo, and thus allow the new tissue to form without the long-term presence of foreign material (Matsumura et al. 2003).

Application of these techniques from the laboratory to the clinical setting have begun, where autologous vascular cells were harvested, expanded, and seeded onto a biodegradable scaffold (Shin'oka et al. 2001). The resultant autologous construct was used to replace a stenosed pulmonary artery that had been previously repaired. Seven months after implantation, no evidence of graft occlusion or aneurysmal changes were noted in the recipient.

3.6.7 Cartilage

Full-thickness articular cartilage lesions have limited healing capacity and thus represent a difficult management issue for the clinicians who treat adult patients with damaged articular cartilage (Hunter 1995; O'Driscoll 1998). Large defects can be associated with mechanical instability and may lead to degenerative joint disease if left untreated (Buckwalter and Lohmander 1994; Buckwalter and Mankin 1998). Chondrocytes were expanded and cultured onto biodegradable scaffolds to create engineered cartilage for use in large osteochondral defects in rabbits (Schaefer et al. 2002). When sutured to a subchondral support, the engineered cartilage was able to withstand physiologic loading and underwent orderly remodeling of the large osteochondral defects in adult rabbits. Thus, the engineered cartilage was able to provide a biomechanically functional template that was able to undergo orderly remodeling when subjected to quantitative structural and functional analyses.

Few treatment options are currently available for patients who suffer from severe congenital tracheal pathology, such as stenosis, atresia, and agenesis, due to the limited availability of autologous transplantable tissue in the neonatal period. Tissue engineering in the fetal period may be a viable alternative for the surgical treatment of these prenatally diagnosed congenital anomalies, as cells could be harvested and grown into transplantable tissue in parallel with the remainder of gestation. Chondrocytes from both elastic and hyaline cartilage specimens have been harvested from fetal lambs, expanded in vitro, then dynamically seeded onto biodegradable scaffolds (Fuchs et al. 2002). The constructs were then implanted as replacement tracheal tissue in fetal lambs. The resultant tissue-engineered cartilage was noted to undergo engraftment and epithelialization, while maintaining its structural support and patency. Furthermore, if native tracheal tissue is unavailable, engineered cartilage may be derived from bone marrow-derived mesenchymal progenitor cells as well (Fuchs et al. 2003).

3.7 Cellular Therapies

3.7.1 Bulking Agents

Injectable bulking agents can be endoscopically used in the treatment of both urinary incontinence and vesicoureteral reflux. The advantages in treating urinary incontinence and vesicoureteral reflux with this minimally invasive approach include the simplicity of this quick outpatient procedure and the low morbidity associated with it. Several investigators are seeking alternative implant materials that would be safe for human use (Kershen and Atala 1999b).

The ideal substance for the endoscopic treatment of reflux and incontinence should be injectable, nonantigenic, nonmigratory, volume stable, and safe for human use. Toward this goal, long-term studies were conducted to determine the effect of injectable chondrocytes in vivo (Atala et al. 1993a). It was initially determined that alginate, a liquid solution of gluronic and mannuronic acid, embedded with chondrocytes, could serve as a synthetic substrate for the injectable delivery and maintenance of cartilage architecture in vivo. Alginate undergoes hydrolytic biodegradation and its degradation time can be varied depending on the concentration of each of the polysaccharides. The use of autologous cartilage for the treatment of vesicoureteral reflux in humans would satisfy all the requirements for an ideal injectable substance.

Chondrocytes derived from an ear biopsy can be readily grown and expanded in culture. Neocartilage formation can be achieved in vitro and in vivo using chondrocytes cultured on synthetic biodegradable polymers. In these experiments, the cartilage matrix replaced the alginate as the polysaccharide polymer underwent biodegradation. This system was adapted for the treatment of vesicoureteral reflux in a porcine model (Atala et al. 1994b). These studies showed that chondrocytes can be easily harvested and combined with alginate in vitro, the suspension can be easily injected cystoscopically, and the elastic cartilage tissue formed is able to correct vesicoureteral reflux without any evidence of obstruction.

Two multicenter clinical trials were conducted using the above engineered chondrocyte technology. Patients with vesicoureteral reflux were treated at ten centers throughout the United States. The

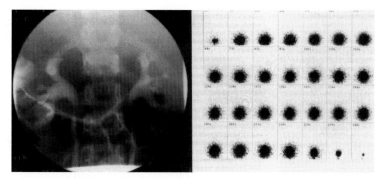

Fig. 4. Autologous chondrocytes for the treatment of vesicoureteral reflux. *Left:* Preoperative voiding cystourethrogram of a patient with bilateral reflux. *Right:* Postoperative radionuclide cystogram of the same patient 6 months after injection of autologous chondrocytes

patients had a similar success rate as with other injectable substances in terms of cure (Fig. 4). Chondrocyte formation was not noted in patients who had treatment failure. The patients who were cured would supposedly have a biocompatible region of engineered autologous tissue present, rather than a foreign material (Diamond and Caldamone 1999). Patients with urinary incontinence were also treated endoscopically with injected chondrocytes at three different medical centers. Phase 1 trials showed an approximate success rate of 80% at both 3 and 12 months postoperatively (Bent et al. 2001).

3.7.2 Injectable Muscle Cells

The potential use of injectable, cultured myoblasts for the treatment of stress urinary incontinence has been investigated (Chancellor et al. 2000; Yokoyama et al. 1999). Labeled myoblasts were directly injected into the proximal urethra and lateral bladder walls of nude mice with a micro-syringe in an open surgical procedure. Tissue harvested up to 35 days postinjection contained the labeled myoblasts, as well as evidence of differentiation of the labeled myoblasts into regenerative myofibers. The authors reported that a significant portion of the injected myoblast population persisted in vivo. Similar techniques of sphincteric-derived muscle cells have been used for the treatment of urinary incontinence in a pig model (Strasser et al. 2003). The fact that myoblasts can be labeled and survive after injection and begin the process of myogenic differentiation further supports the feasibility of using cultured cells of muscular origin as an injectable bioimplant.

The use of injectable muscle precursor cells has also been investigated for use in the treatment of urinary incontinence due to irreversible urethral sphincter injury or maldevelopment. Muscle precursor cells are the quiescent satellite cells found in each myofiber that proliferate to form myoblasts and eventually myotubes and new muscle tissue. Intrinsic muscle precursor cells have previously been shown to play an active role in the regeneration of injured striated urethral sphincter (Yiou et al. 2003a). In a subsequent study, autologous muscle precursor cells were injected into a rat model of urethral sphincter injury, and both replacement of mature myotubes as well as restoration of functional motor units were noted in the regenerating sphincteric muscle tissue (Yiou et al. 2003b). This is the first demonstration of the replacement of both sphincter muscle tissue and its innervation by the injection of muscle precursor cells. As a result, muscle precursor cells may be a minimally invasive solution for urinary incontinence in patients with irreversible urinary sphincter muscle insufficiency.

3.7.3 Endocrine Replacement

Patients with testicular dysfunction and hypogonadal disorders are dependent on androgen replacement therapy to restore and maintain physiological levels of serum testosterone and its metabolites, dihydrotestosterone and estradiol (Machluf et al. 2003). Currently available androgen replacement modalities, such as testosterone tablets and capsules, depot injections, and skin patches may be associated with fluctuating serum levels and complications such as fluid and nitrogen retention, erythropoiesis, hypertension, and bone density changes (Santen and Swerdloff 1990). Since Leydig cells of the testes are the major source of testosterone in men, implantation of heterologous Leydig cells or gonadal tissue fragments have previously been proposed as a method for chronic testosterone replacement (Tai et al. 1989; van Dam et al. 1989). But these approaches were limited by the failure of the tissues and cells to produce testosterone.

Encapsulation of cells in biocompatible and semipermeable polymeric membranes has been an effective method to protect against a host immune response as well as to maintain viability of the cells while allowing the secretion of desired therapeutic agents (De Vos et al. 1997; Tai and Sun 1993). Alginate-poly-L-lysine-encapsulated Leydig cell microspheres were used as a novel method for testosterone delivery in vivo (Machluf et al. 2003). Elevated stable serum testosterone levels were noted in castrated adult rats over the course of the study, suggesting that microencapsulated Leydig cells may be a potential therapeutic modality for testosterone supplementation.

3.7.4 Angiogenic Agents

The engineering of large organs will require a vascular network of arteries, veins, and capillaries to deliver nutrients to each cell. One possible method of vascularization is through the use of gene delivery of angiogenic agents such as vascular endothelial growth factor (VEGF) with the implantation of vascular endothelial cells (EC) in order to enhance neovascularization of engineered tissues. Skeletal myoblasts from adult mice were cultured and transfected with an adenovirus encoding VEGF and combined with human vascular endothelial cells (Nomi et al. 2002). The mixtures of cells were injected subcutaneously in nude mice, and the engineered tissues were retrieved up to 8 weeks after implantation. The transfected cells were noted to form muscle with neovascularization by histology and immunohistochemical probing with maintenance of their muscle volume, while engineered muscle of nontransfected cells had a significantly smaller mass of cells with loss of muscle volume over time, less neovascularization, and no surviving endothelial cells. These results indicate that a combination of VEGF and endothelial cells may be useful for inducing neovascularization and volume preservation in engineered tissue.

3.7.5 Antiangiogenic Agents

The delivery of antiangiogenic agents may help to slow tumor growth for a variety of neoplasms. Encapsulated hamster kidney cells transfected with the angiogenesis inhibitor endostatin were used for local delivery on human glioma cell line xenografts (Joki et al. 2001). The release of biologically active endostatin led to significant inhibition of endothelial cell proliferation and substantial reduction in tumor weight. Continuous local delivery of endostatin via encapsulated endostatin-secreting cells may be an effective therapeutic option for a variety of tumor types.

3.8 Conclusions

Tissue engineering efforts are currently underway for virtually every type of tissue and organ within the human body. As tissue engineering incorporates the fields of cell transplantation, materials science, and engineering, personnel who have mastered the techniques of cell harvest, culture, expansion, transplantation, as well as polymer design are essential for the successful application of this technology. Various engineered tissues are at different stages of development, with some already being used clinically, a few in preclinical trials, and some in the discovery stage. Recent progress suggests that engineered tissues may have an expanded clinical applicability in the future as they represent a viable therapeutic option for those requiring tissue replacement. More recently, major advances in the areas of stem cell biology, tissue engineering, and nuclear transfer techniques have made it possible to combine these technologies to create the comprehensive scientific field of regenerative medicine.

References

Aebischer P, Ip TK, Panol G, Galletti PM (1987) The bioartificial kidney: progress towards an ultrafiltration device with renal epithelial cells processing. Life Support Syst 5:159–168

Amiel GE, Atala A (1999b) Current and future modalities for functional renal replacement. Urol Clin North Am 26:235–246, xi

Amiel GE, Yoo JJ, Atala A (2000) Renal therapy using tissue-engineered constructs and gene delivery. World J Urol 18:71–79

Amit M, Margulets V, Segev H, Shariki K, Laevsky I, Coleman R, Itskovitz-Eldor J (2003) Human feeder layers for human embryonic stem cells. Biol Reprod 68:2150–2156

Assady S, Maor G, Amit M, Itskovitz-Eldor J, Skorecki KL, Tzukerman M (2001) Insulin production by human embryonic stem cells. Diabetes 50:1691–1697

Atala A, Lanza RP (2001) Preface. In: Atala A, Lanza RP (eds) Methods of tissue engineering. Academic Press, San Diego

Atala A, Mooney D (1997) Preface. In: Atala A (ed) Tissue engineering. Birkhauser Press, Boston

Atala A, Vacanti JP, Peters CA, Mandell J, Retik AB, Freeman MR (1992) Formation of urothelial structures in vivo from dissociated cells attached to biodegradable polymer scaffolds in vitro. J Urol 148:658–662

Atala A, Cima LG, Kim W, Paige KT, Vacanti JP, Retik AB, Vacanti CA (1993a) Injectable alginate seeded with chondrocytes as a potential treatment for vesicoureteral reflux. J Urol 150:745–747

Atala A, Freeman MR, Vacanti JP, Shepard J, Retik AB (1993b) Implantation in vivo and retrieval of artificial structures consisting of rabbit and human urothelium and human bladder muscle. J Urol 150:608–612

Atala A, Kim W, Paige KT, Vacanti CA, Retik AB (1994) Endoscopic treatment of vesicoureteral reflux with a chondrocyte-alginate suspension. J Urol 152:641–643; discussion 644

Atala A, Guzman L, Retik AB (1999) A novel inert collagen matrix for hypospadias repair. J Urol 162:1148–1151

Auchincloss H, Bonventre JV (2002) Transplanting cloned cells into therapeutic promise (comment). Nat Biotechnol 20:665–666

Baguisi A, Behboodi E, Melican DT, Pollock JS, Destrempes MM, Cammuso C, Williams JL, Nims SD, Porter CA, Midura P, Palacios MJ, Ayres SL, Denniston RS, Hayes ML, Ziomek CA, Meade HM, Godke RA, Gavin WG, Overstrom EW, Echelard Y (1999) Production of goats by somatic cell nuclear transfer. Nat Biotechnol 17:456–461

Bazeed MA, Thuroff JW, Schmidt RA, Tanagho EA (1983) New treatment for urethral strictures. Urology 21:53–57

Bent A, Tutrone R, McLennan M, Lloyd K, Kennelly M, Badlani G (2001) Treatment of intrinsic sphincter deficiency using autologous ear chondrocytes as a bulking agent. Neurourol Urodyn 20:157–165

Bergsma JE, Rozema FR, Bos RR, Boering G, de Bruijn WC, Pennings AJ (1995) In vivo degradation and biocompatibility study of in vitro pre-degraded as polymerized polyactide particles (comment). Biomaterials 16:267–274

Betthauser J, Forsberg E, Augenstein M, Childs L, Eilertsen K, Enos J, Forsythe T, Golueke P, Jurgella G, Koppang R, Lesmeister T, Mallon K, Mell G, Misica P, Pace M, Pfister-Genskow M, Strelchenko N, Voelker

G, Watt S, Thompson S, Bishop M (2000) Production of cloned pigs from in vitro systems (comment). Nat Biotechnol 18:1055–1059

Briggs R, King TJ (1952) Transplantation of living nuclei from blastula cells into enucleated frogs' eggs. Proc Natl Acad Sci 38:455–463

Brivanlou AH, Gage FH, Jaenisch R, Jessell T, Melton D, Rossant J (2003) Stem cells. Setting standards for human embryonic stem cells (comment). Science 300:913–916

Buckwalter JA, Lohmander S (1994) Operative treatment of osteoarthrosis. Current practice and future development. J Bone Joint Surg Am 76:1405–1418

Buckwalter JA, Mankin HJ (1998) Articular cartilage repair and transplantation. Arthritis Rheuma 41:1331–1342

Campbell KH, McWhir J, Ritchie WA, Wilmut I (1996) Sheep cloned by nuclear transfer from a cultured cell line (comment). Nature 380:64–66

Carrel A, Lindbergh C (1938) The culture of organs. Paul B. Hoeber, New York

Chancellor MB, Yokoyama T, Tirney S, Mattes CE, Ozawa H, Yoshimura N, de Groat WC, Huard J (2000) Preliminary results of myoblast injection into the urethra and bladder wall: a possible method for the treatment of stress urinary incontinence and impaired detrusor contractility. Neurourol Urodyn 19:279–287

Chen F, Yoo JJ, Atala A (1999) Acellular collagen matrix as a possible "off the shelf" biomaterial for urethral repair. Urology 54:407–410

Cibelli JB, Stice SL, Golueke PJ, Kane JJ, Jerry J, Blackwell C, Ponce de Leon FA, Robl JM (1998) Cloned transgenic calves produced from nonquiescent fetal fibroblasts (comment). Science 280:1256–1258

Cilento BG, Freeman MR, Schneck FX, Retik AB, Atala A (1994) Phenotypic and cytogenetic characterization of human bladder urothelia expanded in vitro. J Urol 152:665–670

Colman A, Kind A (2000) Therapeutic cloning: concepts and practicalities. Trends Biotechnol 18:192–196

Dahms SE, Piechota HJ, Dahiya R, Lue TF, Tanagho EA (1998) Composition and biomechanical properties of the bladder acellular matrix graft: comparative analysis in rat, pig and human. Br J Urol 82:411–419

De Filippo RE, Pohl HG, Yoo JJ, Atala A (2002a) Total penile urethral replacement with autologous cell-seeded collagen matrices (abstract). J Urol 167 (Suppl):152–153

De Filippo RE, Yoo JJ, Atala A (2002b) Urethral replacement using cell seeded tubularized collagen matrices. J Urol 168:1789–1792; discussion 1792–1793

De Filippo RE, Yoo JJ, Atala A (2003a) Engineering of vaginal tissue for total reconstruction. J Urol 169(Suppl):A1057

De Filippo RE, Yoo JJ, Atala A (2003b) Engineering of vaginal tissue in vivo. Tissue Engineering 9:301–306

De Sousa PA, Dobrinsky JR, Zhu J, Archibald AL, Ainslie A, Bosma W, Bowering J, Bracken J, Ferrier PM, Fletcher J, Gasparrini B, Harkness L,

Johnston P, Ritchie M, Ritchie WA, Travers A, Albertini D, Dinnyes A, King TJ, Wilmut I (2002) Somatic cell nuclear transfer in the pig: control of pronuclear formation and integration with improved methods for activation and maintenance of pregnancy. Biol Reprod 66:642–650

De Vos P, De Haan B, Van Schilfgaarde R (1997) Effect of the alginate composition on the biocompatibility of alginate-polylysine microcapsules. Biomaterials 18:273–278

Deuel TF (1997) Growth Factors. In: Lanza RP, Langer R, Chick WL (eds) Principles of tissue engineering. Academic Press, New York, pp 133–149

Diamond DA, Caldamone AA (1999) Endoscopic correction of vesicoureteral reflux in children using autologous chondrocytes: preliminary results. J Urol 162:1185–1188

El-Kassaby AW, Retik AB, Yoo JJ, Atala A (2003) Urethral stricture repair with an off-the-shelf collagen matrix. J Urol 169:170–173; discussion 173

Evans MJ, Gurer C, Loike JD, Wilmut I, Schnieke AE, Schon EA (1999) Mitochondrial DNA genotypes in nuclear transfer-derived cloned sheep. Nat Genet 23:90–93

Fauza DO, Fishman SJ, Mehegan K, Atala A (1998a) Videofetoscopically assisted fetal tissue engineering: bladder augmentation. J Pediatr Surg 33:7–12

Fauza DO, Fishman SJ, Mehegan K, Atala A (1998b) Videofetoscopically assisted fetal tissue engineering: skin replacement. J Pediatr Surg 33: 357–361

Fischer Lindahl K, Hermel E, Loveland BE, Wang CR (1991) Maternally transmitted antigen of mice: a model transplantation antigen. Annu Rev Immunol 9:351–372

Freed LE, Vunjak-Novakovic G, Biron RJ, Eagles DB, Lesnoy DC, Barlow SK, Langer R (1994) Biodegradable polymer scaffolds for tissue engineering. Biotechnology 12:689–693

Freeman MR, Yoo JJ, Raab G, Soker S, Adam RM, Schneck FX, Renshaw AA, Klagsbrun M, Atala A (1997) Heparin-binding EGF-like growth factor is an autocrine growth factor for human urothelial cells and is synthesized by epithelial and smooth muscle cells in the human bladder. J Clin Invest 99:1028–1036

Fuchs JR, Terada S, Ochoa ER, Vacanti JP, Fauza DO (2002) Fetal tissue engineering: in utero tracheal augmentation in an ovine model. J Pediatr Surg 37:1000–1006; discussion 1000–1006

Fuchs JR, Hannouche D, Terada S, Vacanti JP, Fauza DO (2003) Fetal tracheal augmentation with cartilage engineered from bone marrow-derived mesenchymal progenitor cells. J Pediatr Surg 38:984–987

Gilding DK (1981) Biodegradable polymers. In Williams DF (ed) Biocompatibility of clinical implant materials. CRC Press, Boca Raton, pp 209–232

Godbey WT, Atala A (2002) In vitro systems for tissue engineering. Ann NY Acad Sci 961:10–26

Gurdon JB (1962) Adult frogs derived from the nuclei of single somatic cells. Dev Biol 4:256–273

Hadley GA, Linders B, Mohanakumar T (1992) Immunogenicity of MHC class I alloantigens expressed on parenchymal cells in the human kidney. Transplantation 54:537–542

Harris LD, Kim BS, Mooney DJ (1998) Open pore biodegradable matrices formed with gas foaming. J Biomed Mater Res 42:396–402

Harriss DR (1995) Smooth muscle cell culture: a new approach to the study of human detrusor physiology and pathophysiology. Br J Urol 75:18–26

Hiendleder S, Schmutz SM, Erhardt G, Green RD, Plante Y (1999) Transmitochondrial differences and varying levels of heteroplasmy in nuclear transfer cloned cattle. Mol Reprod Dev 54:24–31

Hochedlinger K, Jaenisch R (2003) Nuclear transplantation, embryonic stem cells, the potential for cell therapy (comment). New Engl J Med 349: 275–286

Humes HD, Buffington DA, MacKay SM, Funke AJ, Weitzel WF (1999) Replacement of renal function in uremic animals with a tissue-engineered kidney (comment). Nat Biotechnol 17:451–455

Hunter W (1995) Of the structure and disease of articulating cartilages. 1743. Clin Orthop 317:3–6

Hynes RO (1992) Integrins: versatility, modulation, and signaling in cell adhesion. Cell 69:11–25

Ip TK, Aebischer P, Galletti PM (1988) Cellular control of membrane permeability. Implications for a bioartificial renal tubule. ASAIO Trans 34:351–355

Itskovitz-Eldor J, Schuldiner M, Karsenti D, Eden A, Yanuka O, Amit M, Soreq H, Benvenisty N (2000) Differentiation of human embryonic stem cells into embryoid bodies compromising the three embryonic germ layers. Mol Med 6:88–95

Joki T, Machluf M, Atala A, Zhu J, Seyfried NT, Dunn IF, Abe T, Carroll RS, Black PM (2001) Continuous release of endostatin from microencapsulated engineered cells for tumor therapy (comment). Nat Biotechnol 19:35–39

Kaufman DS, Hanson ET, Lewis RL, Auerbach R, Thomson JA (2001) Hematopoietic colony-forming cells derived from human embryonic stem cells. Proc Natl Acad Sci 98:10716–10721

Keefer CL, Keyston R, Lazaris A, Bhatia B, Begin I, Bilodeau AS, Zhou FJ, Kafidi N, Wang B, Baldassarre H, Karatzas CN (2002) Production of cloned goats after nuclear transfer using adult somatic cells. Biol Reprod 66:199–203

Kehat I, Kenyagin-Karsenti D, Snir M, Segev H, Amit M, Gepstein A, Livne E, Binah O, Itskovitz-Eldor J, Gepstein L (2001) Human embryonic stem cells can differentiate into myocytes with structural and functional properties of cardiomyocytes (comment). J Clin Invest 108:407–414

Kershen RT, Atala A (1999b) New advances in injectable therapies for the treatment of incontinence and vesicoureteral reflux. Urol Clin North Am 26:81–94, viii

Kershen RT, Yoo JJ, Moreland RB, Krane RJ, Atala A (2002) Reconstitution of human corpus cavernosum smooth muscle in vitro and in vivo. Tissue Engineering 8:515–524

Kim BS, Mooney DJ (1998) Development of biocompatible synthetic extracellular matrices for tissue engineering. Trends Biotechnol 16:224–230

Kropp BP, Ludlow JK, Spicer D, Rippy MK, Badylak SF, Adams MC, Keating MA, Rink RC, Birhle R, Thor KB (1998) Rabbit urethral regeneration using small intestinal submucosa onlay grafts. Urology 52:138–142

Kwon TG, Yoo JJ, Atala A (2002) Autologous penile corpora cavernosa replacement using tissue engineering techniques. J Urol 168:1754–1758

Lanza RP, Hayes JL, Chick WL (1996) Encapsulated cell technology. Nat Biotechnol 14:1107–1111

Lanza RP, Cibelli JB, West MD (1999) Prospects for the use of nuclear transfer in human transplantation. Nat Biotechnol 17:1171–1174

Lanza RP, Cibelli JB, West MD, Dorff E, Tauer C, Green RM (2001) The ethical reasons for stem cell research (comment). Science 292:1299

Lanza RP, Chung HY, Yoo JJ, Wettstein PJ, Blackwell C, Borson N, Hofmeister E, Schuch G, Soker S, Moraes CT, West MD, Atala A (2002) Generation of histocompatible tissues using nuclear transplantation (comment). Nat Biotechnol 20:689–696

Levenberg S, Golub JS, Amit M, Itskovitz-Eldor J, Langer R (2002) Endothelial cells derived from human embryonic stem cells. Proc Natl Acad Sci 99:4391–4396

Li ST (1995) Biologic biomaterials: tissue-derived biomaterials (collagen) In Brozino JD (ed) The biomedical engineering handbook. CRS Press, Boca Raton, pp 627–647

Liebert M, Wedemeyer G, Abruzzo LV, Kunkel SL, Hammerberg C, Cooper KD, Grossman HB (1991) Stimulated urothelial cells produce cytokines and express an activated cell surface antigenic phenotype. Semin Urology 9:124–130

Liebert M, Hubbel A, Chung M, Wedemeyer G, Lomax MI, Hegeman A, Yuan TY, Brozovich M, Wheelock MJ, Grossman HB (1997) Expression of mal is associated with urothelial differentiation in vitro: identification by differential display reverse-transcriptase polymerase chain reaction. Differentiation 61:177–185

Lim F, Sun AM (1980) Microencapsulated islets as bioartificial endocrine pancreas. Science 210:908–910

Lobban ED, Smith BA, Hall GD, Harnden P, Roberts P, Selby PJ, Trejdosiewicz LK, Southgate J (1998) Uroplakin gene expression by normal and neoplastic human urothelium. Am J Pathol 153:1957–1967

Machluf M, Atala A (1998) Emerging concepts for tissue and organ transplantation. Graft 1:31–37

Machluf M, Orsola A, Boorjian S, Kershen RT, Atala A (2003) Microencapsulation of Leydig cells: A system for testosterone supplementation. Endocrinology 144:4975–4979

MacKay SM, Funke AJ, Buffington DA, Humes HD (1998) Tissue engineering of a bioartificial renal tubule. ASAIO J 44:179–183

Matsumura G, Miyagawa-Tomita S, Shin'oka T, Ikada Y, Kurosawa H (2003) First evidence that bone marrow cells contribute to the construction of tissue-engineered vascular autografts in vivo. Circulation 108:1729–1734

Mikos AG, Thorsen AJ, Czerwonka LA, Bao Y, Langer R, Winslow DN, Vacanti JP (1994) Preparation and characterization of poly(L-lactic acid) foams. Polymer 35:1068–1077

Murray JE, Merrill JP, Harrison JH (1955) Renal homotransplantation in identical twins. Surg Forum 6:432–436

Nguyen HT, Park JM, Peters CA, Adam RM, Orsola A, Atala A, Freeman MR (1999) Cell-specific activation of the HB-EGF and ErbB1 genes by stretch in primary human bladder cells. In Vitro Cell Dev Biol Anim 35:371–375

Nomi M, Atala A, Coppi PD, Soker S (2002) Principals of neovascularization for tissue engineering. Mol Aspects Med 23:463–483

Oberpenning F, Meng J, Yoo JJ, Atala A (1999) De novo reconstitution of a functional mammalian urinary bladder by tissue engineering (comment). Nat Biotechnol 17:149–155

O'Driscoll SW (1998) The healing and regeneration of articular cartilage. J Bone Joint Surg Am 80:1795–1812

Olsen L, Bowald S, Busch C, Carlsten J, Eriksson I (1992) Urethral reconstruction with a new synthetic absorbable device. An experimental study. Scand J Urol Nephrol 26:323–326

Onishi A, Iwamoto M, Akita T, Mikawa S, Takeda K, Awata T, Hanada H, Perry AC (2000) Pig cloning by microinjection of fetal fibroblast nuclei (comment). Science 289:1188–1190

Pariente JL, Kim BS, Atala A (2001) In vitro biocompatibility assessment of naturally derived and synthetic biomaterials using normal human urothelial cells. J Biomed Mater Res 55:33–39

Pariente JL, Kim BS, Atala A (2002) In vitro biocompatibility evaluation of naturally derived and synthetic biomaterials using normal human bladder smooth muscle cells. J Urol 167:1867–1871

Park HJ, Yoo JJ, Kershen RT, Moreland R, Atala A (1999) Reconstitution of human corporal smooth muscle and endothelial cells in vivo. J Urol 162:1106–1109

Peppas NA, Langer R (1994) New challenges in biomaterials (comment). Science 263:1715–1720

Piechota HJ, Dahms SE, Nunes LS, Dahiya R, Lue TF, Tanagho EA (1998) In vitro functional properties of the rat bladder regenerated by the bladder acellular matrix graft. J Urol 159:1717–1724

Polejaeva IA, Chen SH, Vaught TD, Page RL, Mullins J, Ball S, Dai Y, Boone J, Walker S, Ayares DL, Colman A, Campbell KH (2000) Cloned pigs produced by nuclear transfer from adult somatic cells (comment). Nature 407:86–90

Puthenveettil JA, Burger MS, Reznikoff CA (1999) Replicative senescence in human uroepithelial cells. Adv Exp Med Biol 462:83–91

Rackley RR, Bandyopadhyay SK, Fazeli-Matin S, Shin MS, Appell R (1999) Immunoregulatory potential of urothelium: characterization of NF-kappaB signal transduction. J Urol 162:1812–1816

Reubinoff BE, Pera MF, Fong CY, Trounson A, Bongso A (2000) Embryonic stem cell lines from human blastocysts: somatic differentiation in vitro (comment). (erratum appears in Nat Biotechnol 2000 18(5):559). Nat Biotechnol 18:399–404

Reubinoff BE, Itsykson P, Turetsky T, Pera MF, Reinhartz E, Itzik A, Ben-Hur T (2001) Neural progenitors from human embryonic stem cells (comment). Nat Biotechnol 19:1134–1140

Richards M, Fong CY, Chan WK, Wong PC, Bongso A (2002) Human feeders support prolonged undifferentiated growth of human inner cell masses and embryonic stem cells (comment). Nat Biotechnol 20:933–936

Sams AE, Nixon AJ (1995) Chondrocyte-laden collagen scaffolds for resurfacing extensive articular cartilage defects. Osteoarthritis Cartilage 3:47–59

Santen RJ, Swerdloff RS (1990) Clinical aspects of androgen therapy. In: Workshop conference on androgen therapy: biologic and clinical consequences, Penn State Workshop Proceedings. Philadelphia, pp 40

Schaefer D, Martin I, Jundt G, Seidel J, Heberer M, Grodzinsky A, Bergin I, Vunjak-Novakovic G, Freed LE (2002) Tissue-engineered composites for the repair of large osteochondral defects. Arthritis Rheum 46:2524–2534

Schuldiner M, Yanuka O, Itskovitz-Eldor J, Melton DA, Benvenisty N (2000) Effects of eight growth factors on the differentiation of cells derived from human embryonic stem cells. Proc Natl Acad Sci 97:11307–11312

Schuldiner M, Eiges R, Eden A, Yanuka O, Itskovitz-Eldor J, Goldstein RS, Benvenisty N (2001) Induced neuronal differentiation of human embryonic stem cells. Brain Res 913:201–205

Scriven SD, Booth C, Thomas DF, Trejdosiewicz LK, Southgate J (1997) Reconstitution of human urothelium from monolayer cultures. J Urol 158:1147–1152

Shin'oka T, Imai Y, Ikada Y (2001) Transplantation of a tissue-engineered pulmonary artery. New Engl J Med 344:532–533

Shinoka T, Breuer CK, Tanel RE, Zund G, Miura T, Ma PX, Langer R, Vacanti JP, Mayer JE, Jr. (1995) Tissue engineering heart valves: valve leaflet replacement study in a lamb model. Ann Thorac Surg 60:S513–516

Shinoka T, Ma PX, Shum-Tim D, Breuer CK, Cusick RA, Zund G, Langer R, Vacanti JP, Mayer JE Jr (1996) Tissue-engineered heart valves. Autologous valve leaflet replacement study in a lamb model. Circulation 94:164–168

Shinoka T, Shum-Tim D, Ma PX, Tanel RE, Langer R, Vacanti JP, Mayer JE, Jr (1997) Tissue-engineered heart valve leaflets: does cell origin affect outcome? Circulation 96:102–107

Shinoka T, Shum-Tim D, Ma PX, Tanel RE, Isogai N, Langer R, Vacanti JP, Mayer JE, Jr (1998) Creation of viable pulmonary artery autografts through tissue engineering. J Thorac Cardiovasc Surg 115:536–545; discussion 545–546

Sievert KD, Bakircioglu ME, Nunes L, Tu R, Dahiya R, Tanagho EA (2000) Homologous acellular matrix graft for urethral reconstruction in the rabbit: histological and functional evaluation. J Urol 163:1958–1965

Silver FH, Pins G (1992) Cell growth on collagen: a review of tissue engineering using scaffolds containing extracellular matrix. J Long Term Eff Med Implants 2:67–80

Smidsrod O, Skjak-Braek G (1990) Alginate as immobilization matrix for cells. Trends Biotechnol 8:71–78

Solomon LZ, Jennings AM, Sharpe P, Cooper AJ, Malone PS (1998) Effects of short-chain fatty acids on primary urothelial cells in culture: implications for intravesical use in enterocystoplasties (comment). J Lab Clin Med 132:279–283

Steinborn R, Schinogl P, Zakhartchenko V, Achmann R, Schernthaner W, Stojkovic M, Wolf E, Muller M, Brem G (2000) Mitochondrial DNA heteroplasmy in cloned cattle produced by fetal and adult cell cloning. Nat Genet 25:255–257

Strasser H, Marksteiner R, Eva M, Stanislav B, Guenther K, Helga F, et al. (2003) Transurethral ultrasound guided injection of clonally cultured autologous myoblasts and fibroblasts: experimental results. In: Proceedings of the 2003 International Bladder Symposium. National Bladder Foundation, Arlington, VA

Tai IT, Sun AM (1993) Microencapsulation of recombinant cells: a new delivery system for gene therapy. FASEB J 7:1061–1069

Tai J, Johnson HW, Tze WJ (1989) Successful transplantation of Leydig cells in castrated inbred rats. Transplantation 47:1087–1089

Thomson JA, Itskovitz-Eldor J, Shapiro SS, Waknitz MA, Swiergiel JJ, Marshall VS, Jones JM (1998) Embryonic stem cell lines derived from human blastocysts (comment). (erratum appears in Science 1998 Dec 4; 282(5395):1827). Science 282:1145–1147

Tobin MS, Freeman MR, Atala A (1994) Maturational response of normal human urothelial cells in culture is dependent on extracellular matrix and serum additives. Surg Forum 45:786

van Dam JH, Teerds KJ, Rommerts FF (1989) Transplantation and subsequent recovery of small amounts of isolated Leydig cells. Arch Androl 22:123–129

Vogelstein B, Alberts B, Shine K (2002) Genetics. Please don't call it cloning! (comment). Science 295:1237

Wakayama T, Perry AC, Zuccotti M, Johnson KR, Yanagimachi R (1998) Full-term development of mice from enucleated oocytes injected with cumulus cell nuclei (comment). Nature 394:369–374

Wang T, Koh CJ, Yoo JJ, Atala A (2003) Creation of an engineered uterus for surgical reconstruction (abstract). In: Proceedings of the American Academy of Pediatrics Section on Urology. New Orleans, LA

Watanabe M, Shin'oka T, Tohyama S, Hibino N, Konuma T, Matsumura G, Kosaka Y, Ishida T, Imai Y, Yamakawa M, Ikada Y, Morita S (2001) Tissue-engineered vascular autograft: inferior vena cava replacement in a dog model. Tissue Engineering 7:429–439

Wilmut I, Schnieke AE, McWhir J, Kind AJ, Campbell KH (1997) Viable offspring derived from fetal and adult mammalian cells (comment) (erratum appears in Nature 1997 Mar 13; 386(6621):200). Nature 385:810–813

Yard BA, Kooymans-Couthino M, Reterink T, van den Elsen P, Paape ME, Bruyn JA, van Es LA, Daha MR, van der Woude FJ (1993) Analysis of T cell lines from rejecting renal allografts. Kidney Int 39(Suppl):S133–138

Yiou R, LaFleuchuer J, Atala A (2003a) The regeneration process of the striated urethral sphincter involves the activation of intrinsic satellite cells. Anat Embryol 206:429–435

Yiou R, Yoo JJ, Atala A (2003b) Restoration of functional motor units in a rat model of sphincter injury by muscle precursor cell autografts. Transplantation 76(7):1053–1060

Yokoyama T, Chancellor MB, Watanabe T, Ozawa H, Yoshimura N, de Groat WC, Qu Z, Huard J (1999) Primary myoblasts injection into the urethra and bladder as a potential treatment of stress urinary incontinence and impaired detrusor contractility: long-term survival without significant cytotoxicity. J Urol 161:307

Yoo JJ, Atala A (1997) A novel gene delivery system using urothelial tissue engineered neo-organs. J Urol 158:1066–1070

Yoo JJ, Lee I, Atala A (1998a) Cartilage rods as a potential material for penile reconstruction. J Urol 160:1164–1168; discussion 1178

Yoo JJ, Meng J, Oberpenning F, Atala A (1998b) Bladder augmentation using allogenic bladder submucosa seeded with cells. Urology 51:221–225

Yoo JJ, Park HJ, Lee I, Atala A (1999) Autologous engineered cartilage rods for penile reconstruction. J Urol 162:1119–1121

Zhang SC, Wernig M, Duncan ID, Brustle O, Thomson JA (2001) In vitro differentiation of transplantable neural precursors from human embryonic stem cells (comment). Nat Biotechnol 19:1129–1133

4 Bone Marrow Cell Therapy for Genetic Disorders of Bone

E. M. Horwitz, W. W. K. Koo, L. A. Fitzpatrick, M. D. Neel,
P. L. Gordon

Bone marrow transplantation is accepted as an effective therapeutic modality for genetic and acquired diseases of the hematopoietic system. This cellular therapy is based on the principle that bone marrow contains hematopoietic stem cells that can repopulate the blood. Over the past two decades, investigators have recognized that bone marrow also contains mesenchymal progenitor cells that can give rise to a variety of nonhematopoietic tissues, including bone cartilage, adipose, and muscle (Caplan 1991; Pittenger et al. 1999). In principle, then, bone marrow transplantation, as a means of transplanting both hematopoietic and mesenchymal cells, could be used to treat disorders of mesenchymal tissues as well as those of the blood.

Recently, several investigators have reported that bone marrow hematopoietic progenitors, possibly the hematopoietic stem cell, can differentiate to multiple nonhematopoietic cells and tissues, derived from any of the embryonic germ layers, invoking a controversial theory of remarkable stem cell plasticity (Horwitz 2003; Krause et al. 2001; Krause 2002; Wulf et al. 2001). Regardless of whether the bone marrow contains several unique stem cell populations, such distinct hematopoietic and mesenchymal stem cells, or whether there exists a single marrow stem cell with a broad differentiation potential, the range of disorders that could be treated with marrow cell transplantation may be far greater than what is currently practiced.

We found the nonhematopoietic differentiation potential of marrow cells quite intriguing and sought to exploit this extraordinary capacity of marrow cells for the treatment of nonhematopoietic disorders, and we selected osteogenesis imperfecta, a genetic disorder of bone, as our model system.

4.1 Osteogenesis Imperfecta

Osteogenesis imperfecta (OI) is a genetic disorder of mesenchymal cells, characterized by bony fractures and deformities, short stature, and often a reduced life expectancy (Byers 1995; Silence 1997). The underlying defect is a mutation in one of the two genes, *COL1A1* and *COL1A2*, that encode collagen type I, the major structural protein in bone. There is a wide variety in the severity of the phenotype of the affected children. In the most mild form, Type I OI according to the Silence classification (Silence 1997), mutations are typically found in regulatory sequences resulting in decreased expression of one of the two genes and an overall decrease in the amount of normally structured collagen. These mutations may be transmitted by autosomal dominant or autosomal recessive inheritance patterns and the affected children have minimal problems with fractures, no significant deformities, are generally of normal stature, and have a normal life expectancy. In the more severe forms, Type

II and Type III, spontaneous, new, autosomal dominant mutations are typically found within one of the exons so that structurally defective protein is expressed at reasonably normal levels. The protein disrupts bone structure by a dominant negative mechanism. Children with Type II OI exhibit 60% mortality in the first day of life, and 80% mortality in the first month of life. By 1 year, there is >99% mortality (however, a few do survive). Children with Type III OI, the most severe form to routinely survive infancy, have numerous painful fractures, severe bony deformities, and markedly shortened stature. The life expectancy of these patients, historically, was quite short; however, with improved awareness, and improved supportive medical/surgical care, many such patients will live a relatively long life.

The severity of the phenotype of children with OI truly exists along a spectrum, without unequivocal criteria to categorize a given child. Although a genotype–phenotype correlation is approximate at best (Byers et al. 1991; Wang et al. 1993), the specific mutation clearly impacts the phenotype. However, the balance of normal and mutated collagen, in this autosomal dominant disorder, also seems to affect the phenotype (Constantinou et al. 1990). Thus, for a cell therapy strategy to benefit these children, only low levels of mesenchymal engraftment, sufficient to alter the balance of normal and mutated collagen, are required to reduce the severity of the phenotype.

4.2 Overview of Clinical Trials

Our work on marrow cell therapy of OI has consisted of two clinical trials (Fig. 1). The first protocol was designed to investigate whether we could transplant unmanipulated bone marrow and attain mesenchymal engraftment in the bones of the children with severe OI (Horwitz et al. 1999). Then, we assessed whether this marrow cell therapy benefited the children clinically (Horwitz et al. 2001). This study was the first prospective trial of marrow transplantation focused on cells other than the hematopoietic cells. In the second protocol, we investigated whether we could transplant isolated marrow mesenchymal cells (defined as the fibroblastic, nonhematopoietic adherent cells) harvested from the original bone marrow donor and recreate the effects of the original bone marrow transplantation (Horwitz et al. 2002). This later study was the first clinical trial of allogeneic bone marrow mesenchymal cell transplantation.

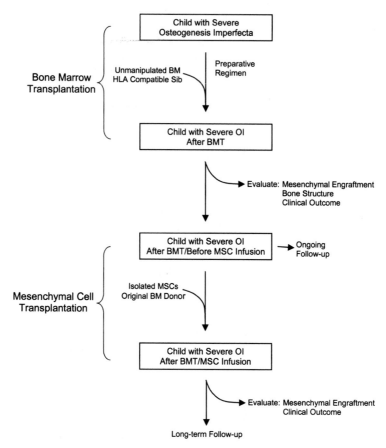

Fig. 1. Schematic overview of the clinical trials of mesenchymal cell therapy for children with severe osteogenesis imperfecta (*OI*)

4.3 Bone Marrow Transplantation

Five children with severe OI (Sillence Type II or III) underwent bone marrow transplantation (BMT) with unmanipulated bone marrow freshly harvested from HLA-compatible sibling donors (Horwitz et al. 1999). There was no unusual or acceptable toxicity among these patients. One child developed sepsis and transient pulmonary insufficiency and another developed acute graft versus host disease (GVHD). There was no other treatment-related toxicity including chronic GVHD.

4.3.1 Mesenchymal Engraftment

Approximately 3 months after BMT, we obtained a bone biopsy from the iliac wing and harvested osteoblasts in the laboratory. After culture expansion of the cells, we verified the absence of hematopoietic contamination and analyzed the osteoblasts for the presence of donor cells. If the donor-recipient pair was sex mismatched, we assessed engraftment using fluorescence in situ hybridization (FISH) for the X and Y chromosomes. If the donor-recipient pair was of the same sex, we used an analysis of the variable number of tandem repeats (VNTR, a DNA polymorphism). Both are standard techniques in hematopoietic stem cell transplantation.

We were able to demonstrate donor osteoblast engraftment in three of five patients ranging from 1.2 to 2.0% of the total number of osteoblasts isolated from the iliac wing biopsy. Although the level of donor engraftment determined in our assay may seem low, we were only able to assess the fraction of donor *osteoblasts*. Bone is comprised of both osteoblasts and osteocytes, the latter being developmental derived from the former. In typical bone specimens, there are tenfold more osteocytes than osteoblasts in bone (van der Plas et al. 1994). Additionally, bone is quite heterogeneous and it is conceivable that the epiphysis of long bones would contain a greater fraction of donor cells than the iliac wing, which is the standard site, and the most surgically accessible, for biopsy in the evaluation of metabolic bone disease.

4.3.2 Bone Histology

If mesenchymal engraftment were to affect the phenotype of the patient, we hypothesized that it should alter the microscopic structure of the bone. Specimens of trabecular bone taken before transplant typically continued numerous disorganized osteocytes, enlarged lacunae and relatively few osteoblasts. The bone had the characteristic appearance of high bone turnover, including woven bone, which is characteristic of OI and other metabolic bone disorders. Fluorescence microscopy with tetracycline labeling showed disorganized formation of new bone and poor mineralization. In contrast, specimens taken about 6 months after transplant showed a reduced number of osteocytes, linearly organized osteoblasts, and evidence of lamellar bone formation. Thus, marrow mesenchymal cell engraftment in the bone is associated with an improvement in bone formation and mineralization.

4.3.3 Clinical Outcome

For the evaluation of the clinical outcome, we assessed three measures: growth velocity, bone mineral content, and fracture rate. These three parameters were chosen because they can be objectively evaluated, and because a therapy that can ameliorate these symptoms would certainly lessen the hardship faced by this population of patients.

Here, we will only consider the three patients in whom we documented osteoblast engraftment. Although we believe it is quite likely that the other children also had osteoblast engraftment and sampling error precluding our analysis from identifying donor cells, definitive proof of engraftment is lacking. Similarly, we do not have definitive proof of nonengraftment; therefore, those patients are inevaluable for clinical outcome.

The patients showed a decreasing growth velocity over the first year of life similar to our controls that were children with severe OI who did not have any specific therapy over the duration of observation. All three patients showed an acute acceleration of their growth velocity during the first 6 months after BMT. Subsequently the growth rates slowed, but remained greater than controls. The patients showed an increase of total body bone mineral content (TBBMC) measured by dual energy X-ray absorptiometry. The rate of gain in TBBMC among these patients slightly exceeded that for weight-matched healthy children and the last few measurements approached the lower limit of the normal range. Although control data is not available for our measurements of TBBMC, OI is a disease of osteopenia; hence, we interpret these findings as suggestive of clinical improvement of bone mineralization. Finally, the rate of radiographically documented fractures acutely decreased during the first 6 months after transplant compared with the 6 months before transplant. Although the rate of fractures gradually declines with age, an immediate reduction in the rate of fractures is inconsistent with the natural history of OI, and most importantly, controls showed a stable rate of fractures over age-matched interval.

This first trial of BMT for children with severe OI represented a significant advancement in the development of cell therapy for OI and other mesenchymal disorders; however, the children were not sufficiently improved to consider BMT, as it is currently practiced, to be a sole, complete therapeutic intervention.

4.4 Mesenchymal Cell Transplantation

In an effort to enhance the benefits observed after BMT, we developed a clinical study to test the hypothesis that isolated, allogeneic marrow mesenchymal cells could be safely infused after allogeneic BMT, and would benefit children with severe OI. To unequivocally identify the marrow mesenchymal cells infused in this trial (compared to cells that may persist after the original BMT) we "gene marked" the cells by transduction with a retroviral vector. Furthermore, to investigate whether marrow mesenchymal cells could be expanded ex vivo, and retain their biologic potential, we used a double gene marking strategy in which minimally processed cells and expanded cells were each transduced with a unique retroviral vector.

4.4.1 Marrow Mesenchymal Cell Processing

After the mesenchymal cells were isolated from bone marrow by adherence to plastic, the cells were divided into two fractions and each was transduced with one of the two retroviral vectors that may be distinguished by a PCR-based assay. One fraction was allowed to remain in culture for the minimal time required for isolation and transduction, while the other was expanded over three passages. The minimally maintained cell preparation was infused into the patients, without a chemotherapy conditioning regimen, at a dose of 1×10^6 cells/kg and the expanded mesenchymal cells were infused at an intended dose of 5×10^6 cells/kg after about 2–3 weeks, again without a conditioning regimen.

4.4.2 Engraftment

About 6 weeks after the cell infusions, we obtained a biopsy of bone, and skin, and an aspirate of bone marrow and isolated osteoblasts, skin fibroblasts, and marrow stromal cells. We then used our PCR assay to assess for engraftment of each cell population. In five of the six patients, we were able to identify marked mesenchymal cells in at least one of the tissues studied. Both minimally processed cells and expanded cells engrafted. Ex vivo expansion may diminish the osteogenic engraftment and/or differentiation potential of marrow mesenchymal cells; however, the limited data in this trial precludes a definitive conclusion of the effect of ex vivo expansion.

4.4.3 Clinical Outcome

All five children in whom we documented mesenchymal cell engraftment showed an acute acceleration of their growth velocity in the first 6 months after the cell infusions compared with the 6 months immediately preceding the infusions. The outcome was most significant for patients 1 and 2, who did not grow prior to the cell therapy, but whose growth velocity accelerated to 94% and 67%, respectively, of the predicted growth velocity for age- and sex-matched children. There was not an unambiguous improvement of the TBBMC after the mesenchymal cell infusions. Since a chemotherapy-conditioning regimen was not given to the children prior to the cell infusions, and the cells were relatively pure compared to unmanipulated marrow (although still quite heterogeneous), the growth velocity data, TBBMC data notwithstanding, formulates a compelling argument supporting the therapeutic potential of marrow mesenchymal cells.

4.4.4 Immunology

Marrow mesenchymal cells have been reported to be immunologically privileged (Bartholomew et al. 2002; Di Nicola et al. 2002; Horwitz 2003; Le Blanc et al. 2003). In our trial, we used two retroviral vectors, one that expressed neomycin phosphotransferase (neo®), and one that did not express the encoded sequences. Interestingly, in all the patients, we found only cells marked with the nonexpressing vector. This suggested that the neo® expressing cells were immunologically attacked when they were infused into these immunocompetent patients. In one patient, we were able to demonstrate, using a chromium release assay, cytotoxic T-cell activity against neo® expressing mesenchymal cells in contrast to mesenchymal cells that were transduced with the nonexpressing vector. Mesenchymal cells, therefore, seem to be subject to an immune response when expressing a foreign protein.

We also evaluated the patients for the antifetal bovine serum (FBS) antibodies, since FBS was a component of the media throughout the retroviral transduction and ex vivo expansion procedures. Using an enzyme-linked immunosorbent assay (ELISA), we demonstrated a greater than 100-fold increase in anti-FBS antibody titers in postinfusion serum compared to the preinfusion serum in the patient who did not show engraftment nor a clinical response. The remaining patients did not show a change in anti-FBS antibody titers after the infusions were completed. Although the lack of evidence of engraftment must be considered inconclusive as detailed above, these observations taken together, suggest that this child had anti-FBS antibodies that attacked the marrow mesenchymal cells, which precluded engraftment and thereby any clinical response. These data further suggest that mesenchymal cells are subject to an immune response when presenting a foreign antigen.

4.5 Developmental Outcome

Although the clinical outcome parameters are critically important to improving the life of children with severe OI, the capacity to enhance their motor development would also be of great benefit and currently there are no therapeutic options. Bisphosphonate therapy increases bone mineral density and decreases fractures, but does not facilitate growth (Glorieux et al. 1998) and may have long-term, as yet undescribed consequences for bone metabolism (Mashiba et al. 2000; Roldan et al. 1999). Surgical correction of bony deformities and placement of intramedullary rods is advocated by many caregivers and seems to be rather beneficial, but this intervention does not decrease the fracture rate nor increase the capacity to walk, which we consider a quite useful skill to improve the quality of life.

For children with OI, several studies have shown that the ability to sit without support at 9 or 10 months of age predicts the patient's ultimate ability to walk (Daly et al. 1996; Engelbert et al. 2000; Wilkinson et al. 1997). In our cohort of six patients, none could sit without support at 10 months of age. Although these children are not yet at physical maturity, two can walk independently, and one can "cruise" around his home. Two children can stand and one has taken some steps, but does not truly walk. The sixth child continues to have significant deformities of his legs so that the bone geometry likely precludes walking at this time.

4.6 Conclusions

Bone marrow cell therapy for nonhematopoietic disorders is extraordinary promising, but such therapy is still in early development. We believe that our work, begun in 1996, has established the proof of principle: bone marrow cell therapy can be applied to nonhematopoietic disorders and especially to disorders of bone. In fact, a recent paper reported that another genetic disorder of bone, hypophosphatasia, had been successfully treated with BMT and a subsequent marrow stem cell infusion (Whyte et al. 2003). Still required, however, are methods that will promote long-term, tissue-specific proliferation and differentiation, thus ensuring maximum clinical benefits from this cell-based treatment strategy.

References

Bartholomew A, Sturgeon C, Siatskas M, Ferrer K, McIntosh K, Patil S, Hardy W, Devine S, Ucker D, Deans R, Moseley A, Hoffman R (2002) Mesenchymal stem cells suppress lymphocyte proliferation in vitro and prolong skin graft survival in vivo. Exp Hematol 30:42–48

Byers PH (1995) Disorders of collagen biosynthesis and structure. In: Scriver CR, Beaudet AL, Sly WS, Valle D (eds) The metabolic and molecular bases of inherited disease. McGraw-Hill, New York, pp 4029–4077

Byers PH, Wallis GA, Willing MC (1991) Osteogenesis imperfecta: translation of mutation to phenotype. J Med Genet 28:433–442

Caplan AI (1991) Mesenchymal stem cells. J Orthop Res 9:641–650

Constantinou CO, Pack M, Young S, Prockop DJ (1990) Phenotypic heterogeneity in osteogenesis imperfecta: The mildly affected mother of a Proband with a lethal variant has the same mutation substituting cysteine for α1-glycine 904 in a type I procollagen gene (COL1A1). Am J Hum Genet 47:670–679

Daly K, Wisbeach A, Sanpera I, Fixsen JA (1996) The prognosis for walking in osteogenesis imperfecta. J Bone Joint Surg Br 78:477–480

Di Nicola M, Carlo-Stella C, Magni M, Milanesi M, Longoni PD, Matteucci P, Grisanti S, Gianni AM (2002) Human bone marrow stromal cells suppress T-lymphocyte proliferation induced by cellular or nonspecific mitogenic stimuli. Blood 99:3838–3843

Engelbert RH, Uiterwaal CS, Gulmans VA, Pruijs H, Helders PJ (2000) Osteogenesis imperfecta in childhood: prognosis for walking. J Pediatr 137:397–402

Glorieux FH, Bishop NJ, Plotkin H, Chabot G, Lanoue G, Travers R (1998) Cyclic administration of pamidronate in children with severe osteogenesis imperfecta. N Engl J Med 339:947–952

Horwitz EM (2003) Stem cell plasticity: a new image of the bone marrow stem cell. Curr Opin Pediatr 15:32–37

Horwitz EM, Prockop DJ, Fitzpatrick LA, Koo WW, Gordon PL, Neel M, Sussman M, Orchard P, Marx JC, Pyeritz RE, Brenner MK (1999) Transplantability and therapeutic effects of bone marrow-derived mesenchymal cells in children with osteogenesis imperfecta. Nat Med 5:309–313

Horwitz EM, Prockop DJ, Gordon PL, Koo WW, Fitzpatrick LA, Neel MD, McCarville ME, Orchard PJ, Pyeritz RE, Brenner MK (2001) Clinical responses to bone marrow transplantation in children with severe osteogenesis imperfecta. Blood 97:1227–1231

Horwitz EM, Gordon PL, Koo WKK, Marx JC, Neel MD, McNall RY, Muul L, Hofmann T (2002) Isolated allogeneic bone marrow-derived mesenchymal cells engraft and stimulate growth in children with osteogenesis imperfecta: implications for cell therapy of bone. Proc Natl Acad Sci 99(13):8932–8937

Krause DS (2002) Plasticity of marrow-derived stem cells. Gene Ther 9:754–758

Krause DS, Theise ND, Collector MI, Henegariu O, Hwang S, Gardner R, Neutzel S, Sharkis SJ (2001) Multi-organ, multi-lineage engraftment by a single bone marrow-derived stem cell. Cell 105:369–377

Le Blanc K, Tammik L, Sundberg B, Haynesworth SE, Ringden O (2003) Mesenchymal stem cells inhibit and stimulate mixed lymphocyte cultures and mitogenic responses independently of the major histocompatibility complex. Scand J Immunol 57:11–20

Mashiba T, Hirano T, Turner CH, Forwood MR, Johnston CC, Burr DB (2000) Suppressed bone turnover by bisphosphonates increases microdamage accumulation and reduces some biomechanical properties in dog rib. J Bone Miner Res 15:613–620

Pittenger MF, Mackay AM, Beck SC, Jaiswal RK, Douglas R, Mosca JD, Moorman MA, Simonetti DW, Craig S, Marshak DR (1999) Multilineage potential of adult human mesenchymal stem cells. Science 284:143–147

Roldan EJ, Pasqualini T, Plantalech L (1999) Bisphosphonates in children with osteogenesis imperfecta may improve bone mineralization but not bone strength. Report of two patients. J Pediatr Endocrinol Metab 12:555–559

Silence DO (1997) Disorders of bone density, volume, and mineralization. In: Rimoin DL, Connor JM, Pyeritz RE (eds) Emery and Rimoin's principles and practice of medical genetics, 3rd edn, Vol II. Churchill Livingstone, New York, pp 2817–2835

van der Plas A, Aarden EM, Feijen JH, de Boer AH, Wiltink A, Alblas MJ, de Leij L, Nijweide PJ (1994) Characteristics and properties of osteocytes in culture. J Bone Miner Res 9:1697–1704

Wang Q, Orrison BM, Marini JC (1993) Two additional cases of osteogenesis imperfecta with substitutions for glycine in the α 2(I) collagen chain. A regional model relating mutation location with phenotype. J Biol Chem 268:25162–25167

Whyte MP, Kurtzberg J, McAlister WH, Mumm S, Podgornik MN, Coburn SP, Ryan LM, Miller CR, Gottesman GS, Smith AK, Douville J, Waters-Pick B, Armstrong RD, Martin PL (2003) Marrow cell transplantation for infantile hypophosphatasia. J Bone Miner Res 18:624–636

Wilkinson JM, Scott BW, Bell MJ (1997) The prognosis for walking in osteogenesis imperfecta. J Bone Joint Surg Br 79:339

Wulf GG, Jackson KA, Goodell MA (2001) Somatic stem cell plasticity: current evidence and emerging concepts. Exp Hematol 29:1361–1370

5 Immune-Based Cell Therapy for Acute and Chronic Neurodegenerative Disorders

M. Schwartz

5.1 Immune-Based Therapies for CNS Injuries

Inflammation, although generally accepted as the body's defense mechanism, has received a bad reputation in the central nervous system (CNS). It should be stressed, however, that inflammation is not a single process, but involves cascades of processes mediated by numerous compounds and factors (Hauben et al. 2000b). The function of inflammation in acute or chronic insults to the CNS has long been a matter of debate. Concepts such as the immune-privileged status of the CNS, as well as observations such as the presence of immune cells in the diseased CNS, have helped to foster the belief that immune activity in the CNS is detrimental (Lotan and Schwartz

1994). Many authors, for example, consider inflammation to be an important mediator of secondary damage (Constantini and Young 1994; Dusart and Schwab 1994; Carlson et al. 1998; Fitch et al. 1999; Popovich et al. 1999; Mautes et al. 2000; Ghimikar et al. 2001). On the other hand, studies have shown that inflammation, by promoting clearance of cell debris and secretion of neurotrophic factors and cytokines, may beneficially affect the traumatized spinal cord. Macrophages and microglia promote axonal regeneration (David et al. 1990; Perry and Brown 1992; Rapalino et al. 1998; Fitch et al. 1999; Ousman and David 2001), and T cells mediate processes of maintenance and repair, thus promoting functional recovery from CNS trauma (Moalem et al. 1999; Hauben et al. 2000a, b).

As more pieces are added to the puzzle it becomes increasingly evident that to describe inflammation as a unified event that is "good" or "bad" for the injured nerve is an oversimplification, because it presupposes a single (and deleterious) process rather than a phenomenon with diverse manifestations. Inflammation is a series of local immune responses that are recruited to cope with the enemies, and its ultimate outcome depends upon how it is regulated.

It is also important to recognize that the beneficial effect of immune activity might not come free of charge, i.e., it might come at the expense of some neuronal loss or transient manifestation of autoimmune disease symptoms. The net effect of inflammation depends on the balance between cost and benefit, a ratio that should be evaluated only at steady state. Accordingly, at certain stages of the inflammatory cascade macrophage activity might be destructive, albeit transiently. This might also explain the neuronal loss observed after injection of zymosan (nontoxic yeast particles used to activate macrophages and microglia) into the healthy rat CNS (Fitch et al. 1999), or injection of encephalitogenic T cells into naive Lewis rats, known to be susceptible to experimental autoimmune encephalomyelitis (EAE).

Thus, the injection of cells or agents that promote inflammatory conditions in healthy animals might cause some tissue loss. The same cells and agents, operating in the traumatized CNS, might promote recovery (Hauben et al. 2000b) and reduce cavitation (Butovsky et al. 2001), and although there is a price to pay (in terms of transient EAE), the cost is outweighed by the benefit.

5.2 Spinal Cord Injury and Immune Intervention

Severe injury to the spinal cord causes irreversible loss of motor and sensory functions of nerves below the lesion, as a result of the hostility of the environment to regeneration of nerve fibers, as well as the poor wound-healing capacity of the mature CNS. In addition to the mechanical, chemical, or metabolic damage sustained as a result of the primary insult, the affected tissue secretes substances in toxic amounts, causing irreparable damage ("secondary degeneration") to neighboring neurons that escaped or survived the initial injury, and leading to further functional loss.

The immune system plays a pivotal role in the healing of injured tissues (Sicard 2002). Injury to the spinal cord evokes an acute local inflammatory response, characterized by activation of resident microglia and infiltration of blood-borne leukocytes (Carlson et al. 1998; Schnell et al. 1999). The inflammatory response in different individuals varies with respect to its time of onset and shut off, its intensity, and its phenotype.

Research over the last few years has shown that there are several local and systemic methods by which the immune response can be boosted or modulated, leading to a more beneficial outcome (Rapalino et al. 1998; Bethea et al. 1999; Bethea and Dietrich 2002; Hauben and Schwartz 2003; Hofstetter et al. 2003). Modulation can be achieved, for example, by incubating autologous macrophages with peripheral nerve segments, thereby transforming them into a wound-healing phenotype, and then injecting these activated macrophages into the injured nerve at the site of the lesion (Lazarov-Spiegler et al. 1998). This procedure was found to lead to significant motor recovery in rats with transected spinal cords.

In developing a feasible therapy for spinal cord injury, autologous macrophages were used as the source of activating tissue. The phenotype and potency of macrophages activated by the skin were tested in a rat model of severe spinal cord contusion, considered to be representative of the human pathology of spinal cord injury. Like the transection model, the contusion model leads to severe paralysis with poor motor recovery in the absence of intervention. To simulate the clinical use of macrophages as an autologous cell therapy for spinal cord injury, activated macrophages prepared from spinally contused donor rats were administered to recipient rats 8–9 days after injury (Bomstein et al. 2003).

The skin-activated macrophages that promoted spinal cord recovery were found to express markers characteristics of antigen-presenting cells (APCs). Recent studies have shown that MBP-preloaded dendritic cells (professional APCs) promote recovery from spinal cord injury (Hauben et al. 2003). It is therefore possible that dendritic cells or the tissue-activated autologous macrophages are acting similarly by providing the damaged tissue with adaptively-regulated macrophages. This is in line with the observations that anti-MBP T cells protect neurons from the consequences of an insult in rats or mice subjected to spinal cord contusion, thus improving recovery (Hauben et al. 2000b). Autoimmune helper T cells were also shown to promote repair of CNS tissue after an aseptic injury but that pathology develops if pathogen-related antigens are present (Hofstetter et al. 2003). Also of possible relevance to the mechanism of action is the ability of skin-activated macrophages to generate brain-derived neurotrophic factor (BDNF). There is evidence that immune cells can be a source of neurotrophic factors (Moalem et al. 2000; Barouch and Schwartz 2002).

5.3 Protective Autoimmunity:
A Physiological Response to CNS Insult

Early studies in rats, using a partial crush injury of the optic nerve or severe spinal cord contusion as a model, showed that systemic injection of T cells specific to myelin-associated peptides reduces the postinjury loss of neurons and fibers. Thus, significantly more retinal ganglion cells (RGCs) survive axonal injury in rats treated with myelin-specific T cells than in rats treated with T cells specific to an irrelevant antigen such as ovalbumin (OVA) or not treated at all (Moalem et al. 1999). Similar findings were obtained for recovery of motor activity after spinal cord contusion (Moalem et al. 1999; Hauben et al. 2000a, b). It was further shown that the beneficial effect of the autoimmune T cells in neural tissue is accompanied by better preservation of the tissue and less cavity formation (Hauben et al. 2000b; Butovsky et al. 2001; Nevo et al. 2001).

In studies aimed at determining whether the observed beneficial effect is a physiological phenomenon, our group concluded that injury to CNS myelinated axons spontaneously evokes a systemic T-cell-mediated response that reduces the spread of damage. In the absence of T cells, recovery is worse (Kipnis et al. 2001; Yoles et al. 2001). Protection occurred even in cases where the autoimmune T cells caused a transient autoimmune disease (Moalem et al. 1999; Hauben et al. 2000a). Interestingly, some strains were less able than others to spontaneously manifest a protective response, a phenomenon that we attribute not to the presence of a destructive mechanism but to the relative impotence of the protective mechanism (Kipnis et al. 2001). Recently, we demonstrated that neonatally induced tolerance to myelin antigens reduces the adult rat's ability to withstand axonal injury, indicating that the T cell-dependent protection which is spontaneously evoked in response to an injury to myelinated axons is myelin specific (Kipnis et al. 2002a, b). Paradoxically, after a CNS insult, strains that are inherently more susceptible to autoimmune disease were more limited in their ability to spontaneously manifest the T-cell-mediated neuroprotection.

This limitation in part reflects the efficacy of regulation of the autoimmune response (Kipnis et al. 2000).

Other studies investigated whether a T-cell-mediated response is spontaneously manifested also after an insult caused directly by glutamate exposure, and if so, whether it can effectively protect the affected site against the consequences of the insult (Schori et al. 2001). Intraocular injection of glutamate into the vitreous of mice resulted in significantly higher glutamate toxicity if the mice were deprived of T cells (Schori et al. 2001). As in the case of axonal injury, strains differed in their ability to withstand the consequences of the insult (Kipnis et al. 2001; Schori et al. 2001). Thus, T-cell deprivation hardly affected the postinjury neuronal loss in strains with low constitutional resistance to glutamate toxicity, but caused substantial loss in more resistant strains. These studies (Kipnis et al. 2001; Schori et al. 2001) provided the first demonstration that local coping mechanisms against glutamate insult are assisted by a systemic immune response. The unexpected observation that the body's immune response can assist the overburdened local coping mechanisms of the CNS led us to extend the traditional view of immune system function as protection against foreign invaders (such as microorganisms) to include protection against the toxicity of self-derived compounds, i.e., against the enemy within (Schori et al. 2001, 2002; Schwartz and Kipnis 2002a; Nevo et al. 2003; Schwartz et al. 2003). The strain-related dependence of glutamate-induced toxicity was found to apply not only to the extent of toxicity but also to the mechanism underlying the toxicity, as shown by the response to treatment with receptor antagonists (Schori et al. 2002).

The discovery that glutamate toxicity is dependent in T cells specific to self-antigens prompted our group to search for a way to boost this response as a means of reducing glutamate toxicity. On the basis of our earlier experience with axonal injury of the optic nerve (Fisher et al. 2001a), the antigens we chose were proteins and peptides associated with myelin. The results indicated, however, that for stress sites containing no myelin, such as the eye (Schori et al. 2001; Mizrahi et al. 2002), this was not the right choice. In retrospect we realized that these antigens could not be effective, because the T cells function only after homing to the site of damage and becoming activated by encountering their relevant antigens there. It was therefore not surprising to discover that the T-cell-dependent resistance to intraocular glutamate toxicity could be boosted by vaccination with antigens that are abundantly expressed in the eye (Mizrahi et al. 2002). An example of such an antigen is R16, derived from the interphotoreceptor retinoid binding protein (IRBP) (Avichezer et al. 2000; Adamus and Chan 2002). This peptide is recognized as a contributory factor in the etiology of experimental autoimmune uveitis (EAU), an ocular autoimmune disease. It therefore seems that a peptide which boosts beneficial autoimmunity at the site of stress is also potentially capable of inducing an autoimmune disease at that site (Fauser et al. 2001). We found that protection from glutamate toxicity in the rat eye is not restricted to IRBP, as two other uveitogenic peptides, both derived from the retinal protein S-antigen, exerted similar protective effects. Moreover, vaccination with IRBP-peptide analogs designed to evoke an immune response without causing EAU also increased RGC survival, indicating that nonpathogenic antigens derived from a pathogenic peptide can be used to protect RGCs from insult-induced death without risk of inducing an autoimmune disease (Mizrahi et al. 2002).

The same principle was found to apply in the case of damage to CNS myelinated axons, where protective myelin antigens [such as MBP or myelin oligodendrocyte glycoprotein (MOG)] were also associated with myelin-related autoimmune disease. In both cases, nonpathogenic cryptic peptides derived from the same immunodominant proteins induced protective autoimmunity without inducing the disease (Fisher et al. 2001 b; Mizrahi et al. 2002). These and other observations support our proposed concept of protective autoimmunity as the body's own rigorously controlled mechanism of repair. More recently, peripheral nerve injury and death of motor neurons were found to be controlled by the same rules and to benefit from immunization with peripheral nerve myelin but not with CNS myelin (T. Mizrahi and M. Schwartz, unpublished observations).

In our view, the threatened tissue endangers some cells for the purpose of saving others. We suggest that the relevant antigen evokes an autoimmune response that, in the event of malfunction, induces disease, but not necessarily in the directly threatened cells such as the RGCs in EAU or myelinated CNS neurons in EAE. Nevertheless, in the absence of appropriate regulation, the autoimmune response might eventually lead to neuronal loss as well. Accumulating information indicates that autoimmune diseases in humans are often accompanied by neuronal loss and an increase in glutamate (Bjartmar et al. 2001; Bjartmar and Trapp 2001; De Stefano et al. 2001; Steinman 2001; Schwartz and Kipnis 2002 b).

5.4 Regulation of Protective Autoimmunity and the Mechanism Underlying It

Our data show that proinflammatory autoimmune T helper cells (Th1) mediate protection against the consequences of CNS insults (Kipnis et al. 2002 a). Thus, paradoxically, the T cells that protect against CNS insults have the same phenotype as those implicated in the pathogenesis of autoimmune disease. The difference in their effects apparently lies in their regulation (Kipnis et al. 2002 b), as well as in the specificity of the response to epitopes within the same protein. Thus, whereas Th1 cells specific to a cryptic epitope (Moalem et al. 1999; Fisher et al. 2001 a) or a modified pathogenic epitope

(Hauben et al. 2001) are protective, Th1 cells specific to a pathogenic epitope within the same protein may be both protective and destructive (Moalem et al. 1999; Fisher et al. 2001 a).

Prior to our studies, the prevailing notion was that the naturally occurring regulatory T cells known as CD4⁺CD25⁺ cells are part of the mechanism that ensures tolerance to self-antigens, viewing tolerance as a state of nonresponsiveness. In our view, tolerance to self-antigens implies ability to tolerate response to self-antigens without developing autoimmune disease. Accordingly, the function of those regulatory T cells is to allow autoimmune T cells (also known as effector T cells) to exist in a state of readiness in healthy individuals for protective action should it be needed (Kipnis et al. 2002 b; Schwartz and Kipnis 2002 a). When protective autoimmunity functions properly (as in strains resistant to injurious conditions), the regulatory T cells apparently allow early selective activation of only those autoimmune T cells that do not carry the risk of autoimmune disease (Schwartz and Kipnis 2002 a). Rats or mice of strains that are resistant to autoimmune disease development, and that are deprived of CD4⁺CD25⁺ regulatory T cells, are better able to withstand the consequences of optic nerve injury than normal EAE-resistant strains. The increase in ability to withstand an insult (Schwartz and Kipnis 2002 a) after removal of CD4⁺CD25⁺ cells is accompanied by an increased likelihood of autoimmune disease development (Shevach 2002). Recent studies suggest that when mice that are relatively resistant to glutamate toxicity receive CD4⁺CD25⁺ cells isolated from wild-type matched controls, they lose the advantage of resistance to the effects of both mechanical injury (Kipnis et al. 2002 b) and glutamate toxicity (J. Kipnis et al. unpublished observations).

Interestingly, the efficacy of the autoimmune response in helping the body to resist cancer development has also been linked to CD4⁺CD25⁺ regulatory T cells. We postulate that regulatory T cells are the cells that determine the risk/benefit ratio, i.e., that they allow a protective antiself response to be manifested without running the risk of autoimmune disease induction. When autoimmune effector cells are needed for protective activity, their switch-on and switch-off is controlled by the regulatory activity of the CD4⁺CD25⁺ T cells. We recently discovered that a stress-related compound produced by the CNS can block the suppressive activity of regulatory T cells, a prerequisite for recruiting an antiself response (J. Kipnis et al. unpublished observations). This compound is a key player in the most upstream event in the cascade of reactions needed to harness a protective response.

In further studies of how the autoimmune T cells display their protective effect, we observed that the microglia appear to act as an intermediary between the systemic immune response and local toxicity. This observation led us to view the microglia as stand-by cells, potentially capable of displaying both immune activity and neural activity as required. This further substantiates our assumption that antiself T cells act as helper T cells (Th1) when called upon to do so. We examined whether microglia, under stressful conditions, can display dual activity, serving both as antigen-presenting cells (in the context of the immune dialog), and as buffering cells (a nerve-related activity). Given our earlier results showing that after CNS insult the injury site is depleted of astrocytes (the usual buffering cells; Blaugrund et al. 1993) and repopulated by macrophages/microglia (Hirschberg et al. 1994; Moalem et al. 1999; Butovsky et al. 2001), this seemed feasible. Moreover, our in vitro studies demonstrated that, like antigen-presenting cells, microglia exposed to activated T cells show an increase in class II major histocompatibility complex proteins and the costimulatory molecule B.7.2, as well as an increased capacity for glutamate uptake (I. Shaked et al. unpublished observations). The effect of T cells on buffering capacity could be reproduced by adding interferon (IFN)-γ (I. Shaked et al. unpublished observations).

5.5 Dendritic Cells: A Therapeutic Immune Cell-Based Therapy Linking Adaptive and Innate Immunity

Recognizing that recovery from spinal cord injury can be facilitated by the boosting of a well-regulated local innate response, we examined the effectiveness of local injection of APCs (in the form of bone marrow-derived dendritic cells) committed to myelin antigen rather than systemic vaccination or injection of blood-borne monocytes activated by the sciatic nerve. We found that the recovery of spinally injured rats injected with DCs pulsed with selected peptides was significantly better than that of noninjected controls.

Since dendritic cells have a short life expectancy within the tissue, local treatment with these cells might have an advantage over vaccination in that they might activate an earlier (immediate) and stronger response, which is local rather than systemic, and is of short duration. As the inflammation required for recovery from spinal cord injury is also transient, this approach is worth exploring for clinical use. The use of dendritic cells to mediate a specific local response is now being explored in other fields, such as cancer therapy. Their possible role in promoting recovery of the injured nervous system represents a new approach.

5.6 A Therapeutic Vaccine for Neurodegenerative Diseases

In designing and developing therapy for acute or chronic neurodegenerative diseases, our approach is based in the concept that a well-controlled autoimmune response, if directed against antigens residing at the site of stress and expressed at the right time, can benefit the stressed tissue without inducing an autoimmune disease.

Our experiments in rats and mice showed that vaccination with the synthetic oligopeptide copolymer-1 (Cop-1; Arnon et al. 1996; Aharoni et al. 1997; Sela and Teitelbaum 2001), apparently results in low-affinity activation of a wide range of self-reactive T cells (Hafler 2002; Kipnis and Schwartz 2002), and can boost the T cell effect, achieving autoimmunity reminiscent of that conferred by cryptic epitopes. Thus, after optic nerve injury or exposure to glutamate toxicity, immunization of rats with Cop-1 protected their RGCs from insult-induced death. This finding suggested that Cop-1 circumvents at least part of the tissue-specificity barrier, and encouraged us to examine whether this copolymer is effective in chronic neurodegenerative conditions (Schori et al. 2001).

As the proposed therapy is based on a concept and not in indications, the same therapeutic approach can be applied in a wide range of indications. As mentioned earlier, the vaccination is directed not against the threatening compounds but against antigens residing in the site of stress. Since Cop-1 circumvents the site-specificity barrier because of its ability to weakly cross-react with a wide range of self-compounds, its use has been extended to numerous models, including head trauma (Kipnis et al. 2003), amyotrophic lateral sclerosis (ALS) and acute motor dysfunction (Angelov et al. 2003), and Huntington's disease (H. Schori et al. unpublished observations).

Studies by our group and others have shown that glutamate participates in ALS, a neurodegenerative condition in which at least part of the motor neuron loss is attributable to a loss of glutamate transporters (Maragakis and Rothstein 2001; Howland et al. 2002). This finding prompted us to examine whether Cop-1 can protect motor neurons in a mouse model of chronic ALS (Angelov et al. 2003). The results suggest that Cop-1 vaccination, in a protocol different from that currently approved and used for patients with multiple sclerosis, can slow down ALS progression, thereby increasing the life span of transgenic mice expressing the human SOD1 defective gene. These results substantiate our hypothesis that autoimmune disease and neurodegenerative disorders are two extreme manifestations of a common risk factor, and accordingly that therapy should be based not on immune suppression but on immune modulation (Kipnis and Schwartz 2002).

5.7 Concluding Remarks

Our findings show that CNS homeostasis is controlled not only locally, but also systemically by the adaptive arm of the immune response directed against antigens residing at the site of glutamate stress. They also provide the first direct evidence that stress-induced immune responses mediate an ongoing dialog between T cells and CNS tissue. As glutamate is a key player in brain activity, and lack of its proper regulation a key factor in cognitive, neural, psychogenic, and neurodegenerative disorders, the novel concept of immune system participation in glutamate regulation might represent a landmark in our understanding of how the body controls the brain and the development of therapies, not only for an excess but also for a deficiency of glutamate.

Acknowledgments. We thank S. Smith for editing the manuscript. M. S. holds the Maurice and Ilse Katz Professorial Chair in Neuroimmunology. The work was supported by Proneuron Ltd., Industrial Park, Ness-Ziona, Israel and in part by grants from The Glaucoma Research Foundation and The Alan Brown Foundation for Spinal Cord Injury awarded to M. S.

References

Adamus G, Chan CC (2002) Experimental autoimmune uveitides: multiple antigens, diverse diseases. Int Rev Immunol 21:209–229

Aharoni R, Teitelbaum D, Sela M, Arnon R (1997) Copolymer 1 induces T cells of the T helper type 2 that crossreact with myelin basic protein and suppress experimental autoimmune encephalomyelitis. Proc Natl Acad Sci 94:10821–10826

Angelov DN, Waibel S, Guntinas-Lichius O, Lenzen M, Neiss WF, Tomov TL, Yoles E, Kipnis J, Schori H, Reuter A, Ludolph A, Schwartz M (2003) Therapeutic vaccine for acute and chronic motor neuron diseases: implications for ALS. Proc Natl Acad Sci 100:4790–4795

Arnon R, Sela M, Teitelbaum D (1996) New insights into the mechanism of action of copolymer 1 in experimental allergic encephalomyelitis and multiple sclerosis. J Neurol 243:S8–S13

Avichezer D, Chan CC, Silver PB, Wiggert B, Caspi RR (2000) Residues 1–20 of IRBP and whole IRBP elicit different uveitogenic and immunological responses in interferon gamma deficient mice. Exp Eye Res 71:111–118

Barouch R, Schwartz M (2002) Autoreactive T cells induce neurotrophin production by immune and neural cells in injured rat optic nerve: implications for protective autoimmunity. FASEB J 16:1304–1306

Bethea JR, Dietrich WD (2002) Targeting the host inflammatory response in traumatic spinal cord injury. Curr Opin Neurol 15:355–360

Bethea JR, Nagashima H, Acosta MC, Briceno C, Gomez F, Marcillo AE, Loor K, Green J, Dietrich WD (1999) Systemically administered interleukin-10 reduces tumor necrosis factor-alpha production and significantly improves functional recovery following traumatic spinal cord injury in rats. J Neurotrauma 16:851–863

Bjartmar C, Trapp BD (2001) Axonal and neuronal degeneration in multiple sclerosis: mechanisms and functional consequences. Curr Opin Neurol 14:271–278

Bjartmar C, Kinkel RP, Kidd G, Rudick RA, Trapp BD (2001) Axonal loss in normal appearing white matter in a patient with acute MS. Neurology 57:1248–1252

Blaugrund E, Lavie V, Cohen I, Solomon A, Schreyer DJ, Schwartz M (1993) Axonal regeneration is associated with glial migration: comparison between the injured optic nerves of fish and rats. J Comp Neurol 330:105–112

Bornstein Y, Marder JB, Vitner K, Smirnov L, Lisaey G, Butovsky O, Fulga V, Yoles E (2003) Features of skin-coincubated macrophages that promote recovery from spinal cord injury. J Neuroimmunol 142:10–16

Butovsky O, Hauben E, Schwartz M (2001) Morphological aspects of spinal cord autoimmune neuroprotection: colocalization of T cells with B7–2 (CD86) and prevention of cyst formation. FASEB J 15:1065–1067

Carlson SL, Parrish ME, Springer JE, Doty K, Dossett L (1998) Acute inflammatory response in spinal cord following impact injury. Exp Neurol 151:77–88

Constantini S, Young W (1994) The effects of methylprednisolone and the ganglioside GM 1 in acute spinal cord injury in rats. J Neurosurg 80:97–111

David S, Bouchard C, Tsatas O, Giftochristos N (1990) Macrophages can modify the nonpermissive nature of the adult mammalian central nervous system. Neuron 5:463–469

De Stefano N, Narayanan S, Francis GS, Amaoutelis R, Tartaglia MC, Antel JP, Matthews PM, Arnold DL (2001) Evidence of axonal damage in the early stages of multiple sclerosis and its relevance to disability. Arch Neurol 58:65–70

Dusart I, Schwab ME (1994) Secondary cell death and the inflammatory reaction after dorsal hemisection of the rat spinal cord. Eur J Neurosci 6:712–724

Fauser S, Nguyen TD, Bekure K, Schluesener HJ, Meyermann R (2001) Differential activation of microglial cells in local and remote areas of IRBP1169-1191-induced rat uveitis. Acta Neuropathol (Berl) 101:565–571

Fisher J, Levkovitch-Verbin H, Schori H, Yoles E, Butovsky O, Kaye JF, Ben-Nun A, Schwartz M (2001 a) Vaccination for neuroprotection in the mouse optic nerve: implications for optic neuropathies. J Neurosci 21:136–142

Fisher J, Mizrahi T, Schori H, Yoles E, Levkovitch-Verbin H, Haggiag S, Revel M, Schwartz M (2001 b) Increased post-traumatic survival of neurons in IL-6-knockout mice in a background of EAE susceptibility. J Neuroimmunol 119:1–9

Fitch MT, Doller C, Combs CK, Landreth GE, Silver J (1999) Cellular and molecular mechanisms of glial scarring and progressive cavitation: in vivo and in vitro analysis of inflammation-induced secondary injury after CNS trauma. J Neurosci 19:8182

Ghimikar RS, Lee YL, Eng LF (2001) Chemokine antagonist infusion promotes axonal sparing after spinal cord contusion injury in rat. J Neurosci Res 64:582–589

Hafler DA (2002) Degeneracy, as opposed to specificity, in immunotherapy. J Clin Invest 109:581–584

Hauben E, Schwartz M (2003) Therapeutic vaccination for spinal cord injury: Helping the body to cure itself. Trends Pharmacol Sci 24:7–12

Hauben E, Nevo U, Yoles E, Moalem G, Agranov E, Mor F, Akselrod S, Neeman M, Cohen IR, Schwartz M (2000a) Autoimmune T cells as potential neuroprotective therapy for spinal cord injury. Lancet 355:286–287

Hauben E, Butovsky O, Nevo U, Yoles E, Moalem G, Agranov E, Mor F, Leibowitz-Amit R, Pevsner E, Akselrod S, Neeman M, Cohen IR, Schwartz M (2000b) Passive or active immunization with myelin basic protein promotes recovery from spinal cord contusion. J Neurosci 20:6421–6430

Hauben E, Agranov E, Gothilf A, Nevo U, Cohen A, Smimov I, Steinman L, Schwartz M (2001) Posttraumatic therapeutic vaccination with modified myelin self-antigen prevents complete paralysis while avoiding autoimmune disease. J Clin Invest 108:591–599

Hauben E, Gothilf A, Cohen A, Butovsky O, Nevo U, Smimov I, Yoles E, Akselrod S, Schwartz M (2003) Vaccination with dendritic cells pulsed with peptides of myelin basic protein promotes functional recovery from spinal cord injury. J Neurosci 23:8808–8819

Hirschberg DL, Yoles E, Belkin M, Schwartz M (1994) Inflammation after axonal injury has conflicting consequences for recovery of function: rescue of spared axons is impaired but regeneration is supported. J Neuroimmunol 50:9–16

Hofstetter HH, Sewell DL, Liu F, Sandor M, Forsthuber T, Lehmann PV, Fabry Z (2003) Autoreactive T cells promote post-traumatic healing in the central nervous system. J Neuroimmunol 134:25–34

Howland DS, Liu J, She Y, Goad B, Maragakis NJ, Kim B, Erickson J, Kulik J, DeVito L, Psaltis G, DeGennaro LJ, Cleveland DW, Rothstein JD (2002) Focal loss of the glutamate transporter EAAT2 in a transgenic rat model of SOD1 mutant-mediated amyotrophic lateral sclerosis (ALS). Proc Natl Acad Sci 99:1604–1609

Kipnis J, Schwartz M (2002) Dual action of glatiramer acetate (Cop-1) in the treatment of CNS autoimmune and neurodegenerative disorders. Trends Mol Med 8:319–323

Kipnis J, Yoles E, Porat Z, Cohen A, Mor F, Sela M, Cohen IR, Schwartz M (2000) T cell immunity to copolymer 1 confers neuroprotection in the damaged optic nerve: possible therapy for optic neuropathies. Proc Natl Acad Sci USA 97:7446–7451

Kipnis J, Yoles E, Schori H, Hauben E, Shaked I, Schwartz M (2001) Neuronal survival after CNS insult is determined by a genetically encoded autoimmune response. J Neurosci 21:4564–4571

Kipnis J, Mizrahi T, Yoles E, Ben-Nun A, Schwartz M (2002a) Myelin specific Th1 cells are necessary for post-traumatic protective autoimmunity. J Neuroimmunol 130:78–85

Kipnis J, Mizrahi T, Hauben E, Shaked I, Shevach E, Schwartz M (2002b) Neuroprotective autoimmunity: naturally occurring CD4+CD25+ regulatory T cells suppress the ability to withstand injury to the central nervous system. Proc Natl Acad Sci 99:15620–15625

Kipnis J, Nevo U, Panikashvili D, Alexanderovich A, Yoles E, Akselrod S, Shohami E, Schwartz M (2003) Therapeutic Vaccination for closed head injury. J Neurotrauma 20:559–569

Lazarov-Spiegler O, Solomon AS, Schwartz M (1998) Peripheral nerve-stimulated macrophages simulate a peripheral nerve-like regenerative response in rat transected optic nerve. Glia 24:329–337

Lotan M, Schwartz M (1994) Cross talk between the immune system and the nervous system in response to injury: implications for regeneration. FASEB J 8:1026–1033

Maragakis NJ, Rothstein JD (2001) Glutamate transporters in neurologic disease. Arch Neurol 58:365–370

Mautes AE, Weinzierl MR, Donovan F, Noble LJ (2000) Vascular events after spinal cord injury: contribution to secondary pathogenesis. Phys Ther 80:673–687

Mizrahi T, Hauben E, Schwartz M (2002) The tissue-specific self-pathogen is the protective self-antigen: The case of uveitis. J Immunol 169:5971–5977

Moalem G, Leibowitz-Amit R, Yoles E, Mor F, Cohen IR, Schwartz M (1999) Autoimmune T cells protect neurons from secondary degeneration after central nervous system axotomy. Nat Med 5:49–55

Moalem G, Gdalyahu A, Shani Y, Otten U, Lazarovici P, Cohen IR, Schwartz M (2000) Production of neurotrophins by activated T cells: implications for neuroprotective autoimmunity. J Autoimmun 15:331–345

Nevo U, Hauben E, Yoles E, Agranov E, Akselrod S, Schwartz M, Neeman M (2001) Diffusion anisotropy MRI for quantitative assessment of recovery in injured rat spinal cord. Magn Reson Med 45:1–9

Nevo U, Kipnis J, Golding L, Shaked I, Neumann A, Akselrod S, Schwartz M (2003) Autoimmunity as a special case of immunity: removing threats from within. Trends Mol Med 9:88–93

Ousman SS, David S (2001) MIP-1alpha, MCP-1, GM-CSF, and TNF-alpha control the immune cell response that mediates rapid phagocytosis of myelin from the adult mouse spinal cord. J Neurosci 21:4649–4656

Perry VH, Brown MC (1992) Macrophages and nerve regeneration. Curr Opin Neurobiol 2:679–682

Popovich PG, Guan Z, Wei P, Huitinga I, van Rooijen N, Stokes BT (1999) Depletion of hematogenous macrophages promotes partial hindlimb recovery and neuroanatomical repair after experimental spinal cord injury. Exp Neurol 158:351–365

Rapalino O, Lazarov-Spiegler O, Agranov E, Velan GJ, Yoles E, Fraidakis M, Solomon A, Gepstein R, Katz A, Belkin M, Hadani M, Schwartz M (1998) Implantation of stimulated homologous macrophages results in partial recovery of paraplegic rats. Nat Med 4:814–821

Schnell L, Feam S, Klassen H, Schwab ME, Perry VH (1999) Acute inflammatory responses to mechanical lesions in the CNS: differences between brain and spinal cord. Eur J Neurosci 11:3648–3658

Schori H, Kipnis J, Yoles E, WoldeMussie E, Ruiz G, Wheeler LA, Schwartz M (2001) Vaccination for protection of retinal ganglion cells against death from glutamate cytotoxicity and ocular hypertension: implications for glaucoma. Proc Natl Acad Sci 98:3398–3403

Schori H, Yoles E, Wheeler LA, Schwartz M (2002) Immune related mechanisms participating in resistance and susceptibility to glutamate toxicity. Eur J Neurosci 16:557–564

Schwartz M, Kipnis J (2002a) Autoimmunity in alert: naturally occurring regulatory CD4+CD25+ T cells as part of the evolutionary compromise between a "need" and a "risk." Trends Immunol 23:530–534

Schwartz M, Kipnis J (2002b) Multiple sclerosis as a by-product of the failure to sustain protective autoimmunity: A paradigm shift. Neuroscientist 8:405–413

Schwartz M, Shaked I, Fisher J, Mizrahi T, Schori H (2003) Protective autoimmunity against the enemy within: fighting glutamate toxicity. Trends Neurosci 26:297–302

Sela M, Teitelbaum D (2001) Glatiramer acetate in the treatment of multiple sclerosis. Expert Opin Pharmacother 2:1149–1165

Shevach EM (2002) CD4+CD25+ suppressor T cells: more questions than answers. Nat Rev Immunol 2:389–400

Sicard RE (2002) Differential inflammatory and immunological responses in tissue regeneration and repair. Ann NY Acad Sci 961:368–371

Steinman L (2001) Multiple sclerosis: a two-stage disease. Nat Immunol 2:762–764

Yoles E, Hauben E, Palgi O, Agranov E, Gothilf A, Cohen A, Kuchroo V, Cohen IR, Weiner H, Schwartz M (2001) Protective autoimmunity is a physiological response to CNS trauma. J Neurosci 21:3740–3748

6 Mesenchymal Stem Cells for the Treatment of Hematological Malignancies

Role in Hematopoietic Stem Cell Transplantation and Bone Marrow Failure

L. Fouillard

6.1 Introduction

Bone marrow consists of the hematopoietic stem cells (HSC) compartment and the microenvironment which regulates hematopoiesis. The microenvironment consists of stromal cells, adipocytes, and osteoblasts, all derived from mesenchymal stem cells (MSC). There is an increasing interest in MSC regarding cell therapy and HSC transplantation (HSCT) for which the main indications are hematological malignancies. MSC are also multipotential stem cells and have a clinical potential in tissue repair.

6.2 Mesenchymal Stem Cells in HSCT

6.2.1 In Vitro and Animal Data

Bone marrow MSC are isolated from bone marrow mononuclear cells (MNC) in flasks in a long-term culture medium where they form adherent cells, get a spindle shape, proliferate, and become confluent. The adherent layer can be trypsinized and then passaged.

Quantitatively, bone marrow MSC represent only one cell for 10^4–10^5 bone marrow MNC. So far, in a regular bone marrow harvest for HSCT, the graft has been shown to contain an average amount of MSC of only 2–5×10^3/kg of patient body weight (Devine et al. 2001).

These cells have a powerful replication capacity in vitro. Some authors reported some time expansions up to 10^{12} corresponding to about 40 generations (Deans and Moseley 2000). So far, from a 20–30 ml bone marrow aspirate, the number of MSC isolated after expansion has been shown to reach 500 million after 21 days of culture (Deans and Moseley 2000), which corresponds approximately in a patient of 70 kg body weight to a MSC graft of 7×10^6 MSC/kg of patient body weight.

MSC phenotype (Deans and Moseley 2000) is characterized by the expression of integrins and adhesion molecules involved in hematopoietic stem cell and T cell interactions. They express the surface proteins SH2 and SH3, as well as the Thy1 antigen. MSC do not express hematopoietic markers CD34 and CD45. Interestingly, the Stro1 antigen defines a subpopulation of MSC precursor. In addition, MSC express the major histocompatibility complex class 1 (Fig. 1).

MSC can secrete either constitutively or after induction by interleukin-1 hematopoietic growth factors as well as lymphopoietic cytokines (Fig. 2). Therefore, MSC are involved in hematopoietic regulation and differentiation, resulting in a pivotal role of the microenvironment to support hematopoiesis (Deans and Moseley 2000). Interestingly, the stromal-derived factor 1 (SDF1) is a chemoattractant factor which improves the homing of HSC and promotes transmigration of $CD34^+$ cells. SDF-1 also acts with thrombopoietin to enhance the development of megakaryocytic progenitors (Jo et al. 2000).

MSC are also multipotential stem cells which can differentiate into osteoblast, chondroblast, myoblast, marrow stromal cells, tenoblast, and

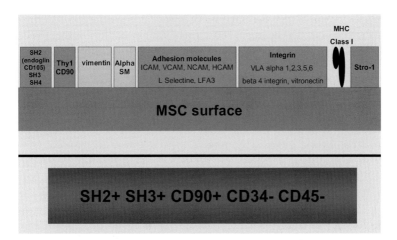

Fig. 1. Mesenchymal stem cell phenotype

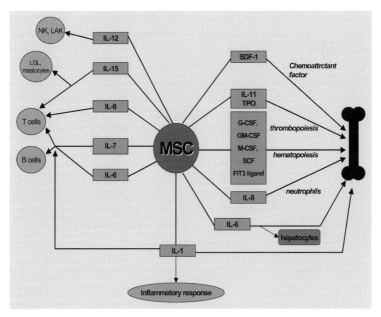

Fig. 2. Expression of cytokines and growth factors by mesenchymal stem cells (*MSC*)

adipocyte (all of mesodermal origin), as well as into cells of ectodermal origin cells such as neuronal cells. This plasticity confers on these cells a large potential in clinics (Pittenger et al. 1999; Prockop 1997).

In a fetal sheep model, this differentiation of human MSC was shown to be specific to the site where MSC engrafted, for example, differentiation into bone marrow stromal cells in bone marrow. This site-specific differentiation was corroborated with a wide distribution of MSC in different tissues, along with a long-term engraftment up to 13 months (Liechty et al. 2000).

In a nonhuman primate model (Devine et al. 2001), systemic infusion of autologous or allogeneic MSC after lethal irradiation was followed by the detection of infused MSC in recipient bone marrow up to 511 days in some animals receiving autologous MSC and up to 76 days in animals receiving MSC from a MHC mismatch donor. This study confirmed the capacity of intravenously infused MSC to establish a long-term residence within the recipient bone marrow.

Stromal progenitor cells can also form a suitable microenvironment to which HSC can home, engraft, proliferate, and differentiate. This was shown in a fetal sheep model where human HSC were injected along with autologous or allogeneic human MSC. The level of human $CD45^+$ cells in the peripheral blood was higher compared to fetal sheep which received HSC alone. This enhancement of engraftment persisted after birth until 12 months and even for over 3 years after transplant (Almeida-Porada et al. 2000). This study showed as well that either autologous or allogeneic MSC were equally effective to support engraftment of HSC.

Promotion of HSC engraftment by MSC was also observed in some NOD/SCID mice model and nonhuman primate model (Devine et al. 2001; Noort et al. 2002).

These studies also raised the problem of cell dose, HSC dose, and MSC dose. First for HSC dose, the study on NOD/SCID (Noort et al. 2002) showed that the most pronounced effect of human MSC on bone marrow engraftment was observed after transplantation of a relatively low dose of human $CD34^+$ stem cells, where with an injected dose of 0.1×10^6 $CD34^+$ cells there was no difference in the level of human $CD45^+$ cells between the group with and the group without human MSC. This finding indicates that in clinics the benefit of MSC could be more suitable for graft with a low dose of HSC.

Then for MSC dose, in a study in nonhuman primate (Devine et al. 2001), hematopoietic recovery following lethal irradiation was faster when higher doses of MSC were infused. In fact, with a dose of 3.6×10^6/kg of MSC, recovery on leucocytes was 34 days; recovery on platelets was not reached. For a dose of 25×10^6/kg of MSC, recovery on leucocytes was faster (10 days) and recovery on platelets was 15 days. This MSC dose effect was more recently suggested in a study presented at the 2003 Experimental Hematology Association (EHA) meeting in Lyon where NOD/SCID mice were injected with two different doses of MSC (1×10^6 and 5×10^6) with CD34$^+$ cells. The level of engraftment indicated by the percentage of CD45$^+$ cells was higher with the highest dose of MSC. Consequently, it means that in clinics the most efficient dose of MSC to be infused in patients needs to be determined.

Beside the MSC dose effect, another concern was that of the subpopulation of MSC according to their phenotype that could be used in transplantation. In a NOD/SCID mice model the stro1 negative MSC fraction had a better ability to support HSC engraftment than the more immature stro1 positive MSC fraction (M. Benshidoum et al., manuscript submitted). This finding may have some clinical applications.

All the studies mentioned above showed that MSC can home in bone marrow and enhance engraftment of HSC.

Interestingly MSC have immunological effects that confer on these cells a particular place in HSCT. Although the class I molecule of the major histocompatibility complex is expressed on the surface of MSC, there is no expression of Class II, Fas and Fas ligand, orcostimulatory molecules such as B7 and CD40. So far, MSC have not been shown to induce a proliferative response when cultured with allogeneic T lymphocytes. In addition, MSC can inhibit T cell proliferation induced by allogeneic peripheral blood lymphocytes, dentritic cells, or Phytohemagglutinin (PHA). The suppression of the mitogen response occurred in a dose-dependent fashion; the inhibition increased with a higher dose of MSC. This inhibition was independent of whether MSC were from the same source as the responder, the stimulator, or a third party (Di Nicola et al. 2002; Bartholomew et al. 2002). Investigation of the mechanism underlying MSC-mediated T cell suppression showed that cell–cell contact was not mandatory. Inhibition was mediated by soluble factors produced by MSC. Blocking studies with anti-TGFβ1 and anti-HGF monoclonal antibodies showed that the proliferative index was fully restored when these two antibodies were used, indicating that these two cytokines, TGFβ1 and HGF, work in a synergistic manner to inhibit T cell proliferation (Di Nicola et al. 2002).

In vivo immunosuppressive activity of MSC was tested in baboons receiving MSC intravenously from MHC mismatch baboon, along with skin graft harvested from the MSC donor or a third party baboon. Prolongation of skin survival from 7 days without MSC to 11 days with MSC was observed whatever the origin of the skin graft. This indicated a nonspecific immunosuppressive effect (Bartholomew et al. 2002). This induction of tolerance was in fact previously suggested in a study wherein a mice model transplantation of allogeneic bone marrow within the donor microenvironment resulted in less graft versus host disease (GVHD) (Gurevitch et al. 1999), and in another study where transplantation of stromal cells in a mice model for autoimmune disease could prevent occurrence of the disease (Ishida et al. 1994).

6.2.2 Mesenchymal Stem Cells for HSCT in Human

According to the in vitro and in vivo data showing that MSC can enhance engraftment of HSC and induce tolerance, the place for MSC in HSCT is very promising:

1. In autologous HSCT to accelerate engraftment and to reduce graft failure, allogeneic MSC being isolated preferably from a related donor.
2. In allogeneic-related HSCT to improve engraftment, to reduce graft failure, and to decrease incidence of GVHD, MSC being isolated from the same donor of HSC.
3. In allogeneic-unrelated HSCT to improve engraftment, to reduce graft failure, and to decrease GVHD, MSC being isolated preferably from a related donor.

There are clinical trials ongoing in North America; a prospective study is being proposed within the association of the European Bone Marrow Transplantation (EBMT) group, and a prospective study will start in 2004 in France within the French Society for Transplantation and Cell Therapy (SFGM-TC).

A pilot study demonstrated the safety of ex vivo expansion and infusion of autologous MSC in 15 volunteers (Lazarus et al. 1995). Then, the same group reported on woman patients with breast cancer receiving high dose therapy followed by a combination of autologous peripheral blood stem cell transplantation (PBSCT) and autologous MSC (Koç et al. 2000). The dose of MSC ranged from 1 to 2.2×10 to 6/kg. Hematopoietic recovery was rapid on neutrophils, but these patients received G-CSF in the posttransplant period. Interestingly, recovery was rapid on platelets with a median of 8.5 days. No adverse event was reported.

In these two studies, autologous MSC were infused. Then, allogeneic MSC were used because of the immunological properties of MSC and because of studies showing that the microenvironment was altered by chemotherapy and radiotherapy in patients.

A phase I study was presented in 2001 at the EBMT meeting by Lazarus and coworkers and reported preliminary results of 30 patients with high risk hematological malignancies receiving a combination of allogeneic HLA-identical sibling HSCT with an escalating dose of allogeneic MSC from the same donor. The dose of MSC was 1, 2.5, or 5×10^6/kg. Hematopoietic recovery was rapid, no graft failure was noted, and 23 patients had no or grade 1 acute GVHD, suggesting a benefit of MSC on the incidence acute GVHD.

In 2002 at the American Society of Hematology (ASH) meeting, phase I and phase II clinical trial results were presented regarding eight patients who received a combination of an unrelated cord blood transplant with MSC transplantation from a haploidentical parent was reported by MacMillan and coworkers at the 2002 ASH meeting. The median dose of MSC infused was 2.1×10^6/kg. Neutrophil recovery was rapid, no graft failure was noted, and acute GVHD occurred in three patients. Despite the low incidence of GVHD and no graft failure, it is difficult to draw any definitive conclusions from this study because of the low number of patients.

Although preliminary results from these phase I and II studies are encouraging, it is obvious that results from prospective comparative studies are needed to evaluate the benefit of MSC on engraftment, graft failure, and GVHD after HSCT.

6.3 Mesenchymal Stem Cells for Bone Marrow Failure

The plasticity of MSC confers on these cells a place in the field of tissue repair and regenerative medicine. Alteration of bone marrow stroma can be induced by chemotherapy and radiotherapy. In addition to the enhancement of engraftment and induction of tolerance, this makes MSC of further interest with regard to HSCT in regenerating a suitable microenvironment. MSC can contribute in repairing a defective microenvironment.

Severe aplastic anemia (SAA) is an autoimmune disease where the stroma usually functions normally. However, damage in the microenvironment has been reported in a subset of SAA patients (Holmberg et al. 1994).

We have reported a patient with a refractory end stage SAA (Fouillard et al. 2003) who received two consecutive doses of allogeneic MSC in order to reconstitute a defective bone marrow stroma, to stimulate hypothetical residual HSC by a local production of hematopoietic growth factor, and to benefit from the immunosuppressive properties of MSC on the autoimmune mechanism of SAA. Bone marrow analyses showed bone marrow stroma improvement and the presence of allogeneic MSC in the recipient bone marrow, suggesting engraftment.

Changes in bone marrow stroma were documented by bone marrow biopsies. Before MSC infusion, biopsy showed no hematopoietic tissue, interstitial hemorrhage, edema, adipocytic necrosis, and no stromal cell as suggested by the absence of positive cell with vimentin immunostaining. After MSC infusion, although there was no recovery of hematopoietic tissue, interstitial hemorrhage, edema, and adipocytic necrosis were not observed and stromal spindle shape cells were visible with vimentin immunostaining.

A chimerism study was performed by real-time polymerase chain reaction (PCR) and was done from two whole bone marrow samples harvested after the first infusion and after the second infusion. The SRY gene primer was used to detect donor male DNA in the female recipient. Presence of SRY gene was detected in whole bone marrow after both MSC infusions. The level of positive signal was low but higher after the second infusion and above the 10 pg control male DNA.

Actually, previous studies in human have already revealed that the level of chimerism of allogeneic MSC was always low, suggesting that a low level of engraftment is sufficient to induce a biological and clinical effect. In humans, detection of allogeneic MSC infused in children with osteogenesis imperfecta did not exceed 1% despite an improvement in growth velocity (Horwitz et al. 1999) and was between 0.4% and 2% in patients with leukodystrophy and Hurler disease despite biological improvement (Koç et al. 2002).

In this patient with SAA it is conceivable that donor MSC engrafted at a low level and then, through cytokine production, recruited recipient residual MSC which proliferated to repopulate the stroma.

The role of MSC in marrow failure including SAA requires further study.

6.4 Conclusion

Allogeneic MSC have a fully therapeutic potential in HSCT and possibly in bone marrow failure. However, there are still some questions. The therapeutic dose of MSC needed in clinics is still unknown. Repetitive infusion of MSC might be necessary to maintain the therapeutic effect and to get a sufficient level of chimerism. MSC are immunosuppressive, can induce tolerance, and decrease GVHD; actually these immunological effects might be deleterious on the graft versus tumor effect. The place of allogeneic MSC from unique donors needs to be evaluated. The place of genetically modified MSC in HSCT also needs to be evaluated.

References

Almeida-Porada G, Porada CD, Tran N, Zanjani ED (2000) Cotransplantation of human stromal cell progenitors into preimmune fetal sheep results in early appearance of human donor cells in circulation and boosts cell levels in bone marrow at later time points after transplantation. Blood 95:3620–3627

Bartholomew A, Sturgeon C, Siatskas M, Ferrer K, McIntosh K, Patil S, Hardy W, Devine S, Ucker D, Deans R, Moseley A, Hoffman R (2002) Mesenchymal stem cells suppress lymphocyte proliferation and prolong skin graft survival in vivo. Exp Hematol 30:42–48

Benshidoum M et al. Transplantation of human bone marrow stromal cells (MSC) into immunodeficient mice. The improvement of human hematopoiesis maintenance and the extent of tissue engraftment depend on the studied MSC subsets. Submitted

Deans RJ, Moseley AB (2000) Mesenchymal stem cells and potential clinical uses. Exp Hematol 28:875–884

Devine SM, Bartholomew AM, Mahmud N, Nelson M, Patil S, Hardy W, Sturgeon C, Hewett T, Chung T, Stock W, Sher D, Weissman S, Ferrer K, Mosca J, Deans R, Moseley A, Hoffman R (2001) Mesenchymal stem cells are capable of homing to the bone marrow of nonhuman primates following systemic infusion. Exp Hematol 29:244–255

Di Nicola M, Carlo-Stella C, Magni M, Milanesi M, Longoni PD, Matteucci P, Grisanti S, Gianni AM (2002) Human bone marrow stromal cells suppress T lymphocyte proliferation induced by cellular or non specific mitogen stimuli. Blood 99:3838–3843

Fouillard L, Benshidoum M, Bories D, Bonte H, Lopez M, Moseley AM, Smith A, Lesage S, Beaujean F, Thierry D, Gourmelon P, Najman A, Gorin NC (2003) Engraftment of allogeneic mesenchymal stem cells in the bone marrow of a patient with severe aplastic anemia improves stroma. Leukemia 17:474–476

Gurevitch O, Prigozhina TB, Pugatsch T, Slavin S (1999) Transplantation of allogeneic or xenogenic bone marrow within the donor stromal microenvironment. Transplantation 68:1362–1368

Holmberg LA, Seidel K, Leisenring W, Storb BT (1994) Aplastic anemia: analysis of stromal cell function in long-term marrow cultures. Blood 84:3685–3690

Horwitz EM, Prockop DJ, Fitzpatrick LA, Koo WK, Gordon PL, Neel M, Sussman M, Orchard P, Marx JC, Pyeritz RE, Brenner MK (1999) Transplantation and therapeutic effects of bone marrow-derived mesenchymal cells in children with osteogenesis imperfecta. Nat Med 5:309–313

Ishida T, Inaba M, Hisha H, Sugiura K, Adachi Y, Nagata N, Ogawa R, Good RA, Ikehara S (1994) Requirement of donor-derived stromal cells in the bone marrow for successful allogeneic bone marrow transplantation. Complete prevention of recurrence of autoimmune disease in MRL/MP-Ipr/Ipr mice by transplantation of bone marrow plus bones (stromal cells) from the same donor. J Immunol 152:3119

Jo DY, Rafii S, Hamada T, Moore MA (2000) Chemotaxis of primitive hematopoetic cells in response to stromal cell-derived factor 1. J Clin Invest 105:101–111

Koç ON, Gerson SL, Cooper BW, Dyhouse SM, Haynesworth SE, Caplan AI, Lazarus HM (2000) Rapid hematopoietic recovery after coinfusion of autologous blood stem cells and culture expanded marrow mesenchymal stem cells in advanced breast cancer patients receiving high dose chemotherapy. J Clin Oncol 18:307–316

Koç ON, Day J, Nieder M, Gerson SL, Lazarus HM, Krivit W (2002) Allogeneic mesenchymal stem cell infusion for the treatment of metachromatic leukodystrophy (MLD) and Hurler syndrome (MPS-IH). Bone Marrow Transplant 30:215–222

Lazarus HM, Haynesworth SE, Gerson SL, Rosenthal NS, Caplan AI (1995) Ex vivo expansion and subsequent infusion of bone marrow-derived stromal progenitor cells (mesenchymal progenitor cells): implication for therapeutic use. Bone Marrow Transplant 16:557–564

Liechty KW, MacKenzie TC, Shaaban AF, Radu A, Moseley AM, Deans R, Marshak DR, Flake AW (2000) Human mesenchymal stem cells engraft and demonstrate site-specific differentiation after in utero transplantation in sheep. Nat Med 6:1282–1286

Noort WA, Kruisselbrink AB, in't Anker PS, Kruger M, van Bezooijen RL, de Paus RA, Heemskerk MH, Lowik CW, Falkenburg JH, Willemze R, Fibbe WE (2002) Mesenchymal stem cells promote engraftment of human umbilical cord blood derived CD34$^+$ cells in NOD-SCID mice. Exp Hematol 30:870–878

Pittenger MF, Mackay AM, Beck SC, Jaiswal RK, Douglas R, Mosca JD, Moorman MA, Simonetti DW, Craig S, Marshak DR (1999) Multilineage potential of adult human mesenchymal stem cells. Science 284:143–147

Prockop DJ (1997) Marrow stromal cells as stem cells for nonhematopoietic tissues. Science 276:71–73

7 Perspectives in Transfusion Medicine for the Ex Vivo Control of Hematopoiesis

L. Douay

7.1 In Vitro Control of the Proliferation and Differentiation of Hematopoietic Stem Cells

The recent development of techniques permitting the selection of hematopoietic progenitors and our knowledge of the growth factors specifically involved in the proliferation of certain cell lines have made it possible to envisage the ex vivo production of hematopoietic cell populations for grafting or transfusion purposes (white cells, megakaryocyte and erythroid precursors). These cells can in fact be amplified through the proliferation of a very small number of stem cells from blood, bone marrow, or placenta.

Over the past few years, considerable interest has emerged for the expansion of hematopoietic cells (Emerson 1996). The field of application is potentially vast:

1. Either to increase the number of primitive stem cells in grafts containing insufficient numbers of these cells, as is the case for cord blood grafts in adults, or to reduce the quantity of cytapheresis stem cells required when their grafting is proposed as a purge in hemopathies and certain cancers; the objective here is clearly to amplify the primitive compartment.
2. Or to increase the number of mature cells in order to reduce the duration of aplasia; the objective is then to induce a massive differentiation of the progenitor compartments.
3. Or to produce cells of specific lineages like megakaryocytes or erythroid precursors.

In this regard, cord blood presents certain advantages with respect to the two other sources: it contains sufficient hematopoietic progenitors (Broxmeyer et al. 1992) to enable successful grafting in children (Gluckman et al. 1989; Kurtzberg et al. 1996) and sometimes in adults (Laporte et al. 1996), while these progenitors give rise to larger colonies in vitro (Broxmeyer et al. 1991) and have a greater expansion capacity (Mayani et al. 1993).

Dexter et al. (1981) were the first to discover a possibility of erythroid differentiation in a long-term murine culture system in the presence of anemic mouse serum. Chelucci et al. (1995) obtained a similar result in cultures of purified stem cells using high concentrations of EPO and low concentrations of GM-CSF and IL-3, but nevertheless without achieving the final differentiation of enucleated erythrocytes.

Malik et al. (1998) have developed a model of human erythrocyte production in sickle cell disease patients based on the expansion of hematopoietic stem cells (HSC) from cord blood, bone marrow, and peripheral blood. The hemoglobin present in the cells amplified from CD34$^+$ bone marrow cells was of adult or neonatal type with β chains and a very small proportion of γ chains after 18–21 days of culture. When 10^5 CD34$^+$ cells/ml were cultured in IMDM medium in the presence of 10 U/ml EPO, 0.001 ng/ml GM-CSF, and 0.01 U/ml IL-3, under 5% CO_2 at 37 °C, a population strongly enriched in reticulocytes and erythrocytes was obtained but with a low level of amplification. According to the authors, this model is intended for study of the physiopathology of hemoglobinopathies.

Freyssinier et al. (1999) have more recently established a protocol allowing the expansion in large numbers of a pure population of erythroid progenitors from cord or peripheral blood in three purification and amplification steps. This protocol is based on an initial 7-day culture of HSC in the presence of an IL-3/IL-6/SCF cytokine cocktail, subsequent purification of the CD36$^+$ early erythroid progenitors produced in culture, and finally secondary culture of the purified CD36$^+$ progenitors in the presence of an IL-3/IL-6/SCF/EPO cocktail. After 7 days of secondary culture, these authors obtained a population of erythroblasts and enucleated erythrocytes. The accession to a purified, amplified population of erythroid progenitors, demonstrated by this group, represents a valuable tool for study of the normal regulation of erythropoiesis.

Our team has developed a procedure for the in vitro amplification of erythrocyte precursors from CD34$^+$ HSC derived from cord blood (Neildez-Nguyen et al. 2002). The cells are cultured in a specific medium according to a three-step amplification protocol: a first step from day 0 to day 7 in the presence of 3 cytokines, *stem cell factor* (SCF), Flt3 ligand, and thrombopoietin, chosen to stimulate the proliferation of primitive stem cells, followed by a second step also of 7 days in the presence of EPO, *insulin growth factor-1* (IGF-1) and SCF, cytokines targeting the erythroid progenitors, and a third step as of day 15, in the presence of EPO and IGF-1, which promote the differentiation of erythroid precursors. After 17 days of culture, the increase in the number of cells with respect to day 0 reaches on an average 200,000-fold (50,000–280,000), with 96% of the cells being erythroblast precursors and 4% reticulocytes. These culture conditions selectively amplify the erythroid progenitor compartment at the beginning of culture, as shown by the peak in the number of these progenitors (*colony-forming unit-erythroid*, CFU-E) at day 10, a peak which diminishes progressively to become undetectable by day 17. The hemoglobin produced under such conditions is mainly of fetal type and completely functional with regard to the capture and release of oxygen. However, although the expansion obtained in vitro reaches considerable levels, the small proportion of enucleated cells is not compatible with the desired therapeutic application.

Different complementary assays have concerned the physicochemical conditions during culture. The proliferation and differentiation of erythrocytes can in fact be influenced by variations in the pH of the medium (McAdams et al. 1996, 1997). Thus, a low pH (7.1) increases the clonogenic capacity of BFU-E by ninefold relative to a pH of 7.6 and fluctuations of as little as 0.2 units above physiological levels are deleterious. The erythroid differentiation therefore increases between pH values of 6.95 (no colonies) and 7.6 (maximum hemoglobinization). The oxygen concentration is another critical parameter which alters the effects of growth factors on the myeloid lineages (Laluppa et al. 1998) and, for example, 2.5 times more hemoglobinized cells are produced in the presence of EPO under a 20% as compared to a 5% oxygen atmosphere.

Hence, whatever the approach considered, none as yet permits one to obtain in vitro at the same time a very high level of amplification of the progenitors/precursors and an almost total terminal enucleation.

7.2 Enucleation:
A Complex and Poorly Understood Phenomenon

During their maturation, erythroblast precursors present specific morphological and biochemical characteristics. A study of immature murine erythroblasts infected with Friend virus has reproduced this differentiation in vitro (Koury and Bondurant 1992). Successively, one may distinguish proerythroblasts with a large nucleus and nucleoli, basophilic erythroblasts presenting a condensed nuclear chromatin and less clearly visible nucleoli, polychromatophilic type I and II erythroblasts in which the nucleoli are practically invisible, reticulocytes, and finally erythrocytes. Cells on the point of enucleation have an excentric nucleus and display an accumulation of hemoglobin, while the free nuclei are surrounded by a thin layer of cytoplasm and generally an intact plasma membrane.

The process of enucleation and thus the final stage of maturation leading to the formation of red blood cells has not been described to date. This complex mechanism involves a certain number of elements susceptible to be controlled in cultures in vitro.

7.2.1 Macrophages and Emp-1 Protein

In the bone marrow the erythroblasts are located in clumps around macrophages. The latter are in close contact with each erythroblast through pseudopods and the entire clump forms an erythroblast island. The macrophages phagocyte the nuclei expelled during maturation of the erythroblasts. These erythroblast islands have been reproduced in vitro from peripheral blood cells cultured in the presence of EPO and of medium conditioned with the lineage 5637 (Hanspal and Hanspal 1994; Hanspal et al. 1998). After 4–5 days, the erythroblast clusters are harvested and recultured and during this second phase of culture, erythroblast islands appear (7–8 days). After 7–10 days, the cells surrounding the macrophages are at the proerythroblast, basophilic normoblast stage. After 12–13 days, one observes late erythroblasts with a majority of benzidine-positive cells, while enucleation occurs after 14 days of this secondary culture.

The importance of the macrophage/erythroblast contact has been well demonstrated in this system. In fact, in the absence of macrophages, the number of erythroblasts diminishes and these cells differentiate but do not enucleate. Moreover, the cell proliferation and maturation are reduced in the presence of conditioned medium alone. This contact involves in particular the protein Emp-1, which is expressed by both macrophages and erythroblasts and enables their homophilic adherence. Emp-1 is specific for macrophage/erythroblast attachment but can bind to heparin. The enucleation of cord blood erythroblasts has been observed in cultures containing erythroblast islands and it can occur in the presence of GM-CSF. It is nevertheless not possible to envisage the presence of macrophages in a product destined for transfusion, although addition of Emp-1 protein might allow one to "mimic" the contact with macrophages.

7.2.2 TGFβ-1

Whereas TGFβ-1 has a negative impact on early erythropoiesis (BFU-E and CFU-E), it plays a positive role in terminal maturation. Its effect has been demonstrated in cultures of the erythrocyte lineage UT-7 whose growth is dependent on erythropoietin (Zermati et al. 2000a). If TGFβ-1 is added to the culture medium, it increases the formation of hemoglobinized cells in the presence of EPO. Its action does not however involve the erythropoietin pathway. A study performed in CD36$^+$ cells selected after amplification has likewise revealed an influence of TGFβ-1 on cell maturation (Zermati et al. 2000b). Although it slows the proliferation of these cells, it accelerates and increases their erythrocyte differentiation (more rapid expression of GPA, appearance of hemoglobin, enucleation). TGFβ-1 could be used to promote the enucleation of erythroblasts in vitro. Nevertheless, in view of its deleterious effect on cell growth and viability, it should be added after cell expansion.

7.2.3 Fibronectin

Erythrocytes are able to adhere to fibronectin, a protein of the extracellular matrix synthesized by stromal cells (Patel and Lodish 1986). This adhesion is indispensable for the maturation of murine erythroleukemic cells (Patel and Lodish 1987). The fibronectin receptors, VLA-4 and VLA-5, are expressed by immature human erythroblast precursors (Rosemblatt et al. 1991) and the importance of the adhesion of erythroid precursors to fibronectin has been demonstrated in vivo (Hamamura et al. 1996) and in vitro (Davies and Lux 1989). Since erythroblasts continue to express the fibronectin receptors up until the reticulocyte stage, it would seem logical that their adhesion to this protein should form part of the final maturation process. Thus, in order to promote the enucleation of erythroblasts generated in vitro, it would probably be of interest to culture the cells on a matrix of fibronectin. Our culture system nevertheless requires heparin and binding of this protein to fibronectin would prevent adhesion of erythroblasts to the matrix.

7.2.4 The Cytoskeleton

The cytoskeleton is rearranged during enucleation and certain proteins play an important role in its organization and in ensuring the plasticity of the cells (for a review see Davies and Lux 1989). Spectrin is responsible for the flexibility of the erythrocyte membrane. The latter contains two glycoproteins which associate with the cytoskeleton: protein 3 (an anionic transporter) and glycophorin C. The cytoplasmic domain of protein 3 is linked to ankryn, itself linked to β-spectrin, while the cytoplasmic tail of this protein can also bind to hemoglobin. Glycophorin C is linked through protein 4.1 to the complex spectrin/actin/protein 4.1. Culture of MEL cells on fibronectin enhances the expression of band 3 protein, spectrin, and ankyrin (Davies and Lux 1989). After enucleation, these proteins are sequestered in the cytoplasm of reticulocytes and likewise of normal erythroblasts. A study performed in human erythroblasts describes well the distribution and possible functions of some of these proteins in the course of maturation and enucleation (Koury and Bondurant 1992). During enucleation, a very intense labeling is visible between the nucleus and reticulum. Spectrin is still found in the cytoplasm of mature cells and remains associated with the plasma membrane of reticulocytes, while filamentary actin (F-actin) is also present in the mature cytoplasm. Use of drugs interfering with these proteins has shown that only F-actin is involved in enucleation.

7.3 In Vivo Fate of the Erythroblast Precursors Produced In Vitro

Since erythroid precursors are incapable, under certain conditions in vitro, of continuing their maturation as far as the production of enucleated red blood cells, we determined the fate of these populations after their transfusion in vivo into *nonobese diabetic severe combined immunodeficient* (NOD/SCID) mice, an animal model classically used to analyze the in vivo reconstitution of human HSC (Neildez-Nguyen et al. 2002). It was decided to graft the cells obtained on day 10 of culture, which consist of 93% of erythroid precursors but still have a high proliferative capacity, as shown by their large content of CFU-E. Grafts containing 30×10^6 cells, previously incubated with the fluorescent marker *carboxyfluorescein succinyl ethanolamine* (CFSE), were transfused into sublethally irradiated NOD/SCID mice. The following observations were made:

1. CFSE$^+$ cells were detectable in the liver, spleen, bone marrow, lungs and blood of the animals, but were not destroyed in the liver or spleen.
2. In the blood, they completed in 4 days their terminal maturation into enucleated red blood cells, a maturation which was accompanied by amplification of the number of cells by about 100-fold.
3. The enucleated CFSE$^+$ cells were erythrocytes expressing the D antigen of the Rhesus system, like those of the cord blood from which the initial CD34$^+$ cells were derived.
4. The hemoglobin present in these red blood cells was of adult type and perfectly functional. One may conclude in simple terms from this model that these precursors had found in vivo the conditions permitting their concomitant proliferation and enucleation.

7.4 A Quantitative Challenge for Use in Transfusion

In this aim of producing red blood cells by cell culture, the objective today is undoubtedly to attempt to combine two properties: the high proliferative capacity of cord blood HSC and the aptitude of erythroid precursors derived from bone marrow to complete in vitro their final maturation into enucleated erythrocytes.

One may already envisage a clinical application of the erythroid precursors produced according to the protocol described above. Thus:
1. 10^6 CD34$^+$ cells (corresponding to 1/4 or 1/3 of the content in the blood collected from a standard umbilical cord vein) are capable of producing $5–10 \times 10^9$ erythroid precursors, which will subsequently continue their amplification and differentiation in vivo after transfusion to reach a total of $5–10 \times 10^{11}$ red blood cells, equivalent to 3–5 times the normal daily quantity synthesized in humans.
2. The transfusion of erythroid precursors produced ex vivo from CD34$^+$ cord blood cells could provide a transfusion support comparable to that of standard red blood cell concentrates (RBCC). In fact, if one considers that an RBCC contains an average of 2×10^{12} erythrocytes and increases hemoglobin levels in the receiver by an average of 1 g, one may estimate as $1–2 \times 10^{10}$ the number of erythrocyte precursors to be transfused to obtain an increase in hemoglobin of 0.5–1 g in the receiver.

3. The production of several red blood cell units from a single cord blood donation would reduce the risks of contamination by viruses or nonconventional agents.
4. Cord blood is a readily available source of HSC.

This work therefore proposes a new technology for the large scale production of erythroid cells which has potential interest for transfusion purposes, insofar as it has been shown for the first time that erythroid precursors generated ex vivo in large quantities conserve a capacity to terminate their maturation in vivo to reach the stage of mature red blood cells containing functional adult hemoglobin.

If these results are confirmed in humans, in other words if these nucleated erythroid precursors are not destroyed in the spleen or liver of the receivers, one could then envisage the constitution of banks of cord blood for the production of red blood cells of particular phenotypes. There exist in fact, in transfusion medicine, situations which cannot be resolved due to the nonavailability of compatible erythrocyte units, due to a complex polyimmunization of the receiver.

The transfusion of erythroblast precursors would have several advantages:

1. *At the level of transfusion efficacy,* the injection of cells which will give rise within a few days to a population of red blood cells homogeneous in age could significantly improve the transfusion rhythm and in the long term decrease the iron overload of polytransfused patients by reducing the number of transfusions.
2. *At the level of transfusion safety,* cord blood presents an obvious advantage as it is less susceptible to be contaminated by viruses which are not systematically tested (EBV, CMV, B19), or by emerging agents whose transmission in the blood remains hypothetical.
3. *At the level of transfusion indications,* one may reasonably envisage the development of cord blood banks for rare phenotypes.
4. *At the level of the perspectives,* this study phase using cord blood is a preliminary stage indispensable for the future development of systems using peripheral blood stem cells for autologous applications.

It is not intended here to propose an alternative to classical transfusion, but rather a complementary approach which now requires evaluation of its feasibility and interest in transfusion medicine for future therapeutic applications, while awaiting the day when it will probably be possible to produce authentic red blood cells.

References

Broxmeyer HE, Carow C, Hangoc G, Hendrie PC, Cooper S (1991) Hematopoietic stem and progenitor cells in human umbilical cord blood. Hum Gene Transfer 219:95–102

Broxmeyer HE, Hangoc G, Cooper S (1992) Growth characteristics and expansion of human umbilical cord blood and estimation of its potential for transplantation in adults. Proc Natl Acad Sci 89:4109–4113

Chelucci C, Hassan HJ, Locardi C, Bulgarini D, Pelosi E, Mariani G, Testa U, Federico M, Valtieri M, Peschle C (1995) In vitro human immunodeficiency virus-1 infection of purified hematopoietic progenitors in single-cell culture. Blood 85:1181–1187

Davies KA, Lux SE (1989) Hereditary disorders of the red cell membrane skeleton. Trends Genet 5:222–227

Dexter TM, Testa NG, Allen TD, Rutherford T, Scolnick E (1981) Molecular and cell biologic aspects of erythropoiesis in long term bone marrow cultures. Blood 58:699–707

Emerson SG (1996) Ex vivo expansion of hematopoietic precursors, progenitors, and stem cells: the next generation of cellular therapeutics. Blood 87:3082–3088

Freyssinier JM, Lecoq-Lafon C, Amsellem S, Picard F, Ducrocq R, Mayeux P, Lacombe C, Fichelson S (1999) Purification, amplification and characterization of a population of human erythroid progenitors. Br J Haematol 106:912–922

Gluckman E, Broxmeyer HA, Auerbach AD, et al. (1989) Hematopoietic reconstitution in a patient with Fanconi's anemia by means of umbilical-cord blood from an HLA-identical sibling. N Engl J Med 321:1174–1178

Hamamura K, Matsuda H, Takeuchi Y, Habu S, Yagita H, Okumura K (1996) A critical role of VLA-4 in erythropoiesis in vivo. Blood 87:2513–2517

Hanspal M, Hanspal JS (1994) The association of erythroblasts with macrophages promotes erythroid proliferation and maturation: a 30-kD heparin-binding protein is involved in this contact. Blood 84:3494–3504

Hanspal M, Smockova Y, Uong Q (1998) Molecular identification and functional characterization of a novel protein that mediates the attachment of erythroblasts to macrophages. Blood 92:2940–2950

Koury MJ, Bondurant MC (1992) The molecular mechanism of erythropoietin action. Eur J Biochem 210:649–663

Kurtzberg J, Laughlin M, Graham ML, et al. (1996) Placental blood as a source of hematopoietic stem cells for transplantation into unrelated recipients. N Engl J Med 335:157–166

Laluppa JA, Papoutsakis ET, Miller WM (1998) Oxygen tension alters the effects of cytokines on the megakaryocyte, erythrocyte, and granulocyte lineages. Exp Hematol 26:835–843

Laporte JP, Gorin NC, Rubinstein P, et al. (1996) Cord-blood transplantation from an unrelated donor in an adult with chronic myelogenous leukemia. N Engl J Med 335:167–170

Malik P, Fisher TC, Barsky LL, Zeng L, Izadi P, Hiti AL, Weinberg KI, Coates TD, Meiselman HJ, Kohn DB (1998) An in vitro model of human red blood cell production from hematopoietic progenitor cells. Blood 91:2664–2671

Mayani H, Dragowska W, Lansdorp PM (1993) Cytokine-induced selective expansion and maturation of erythroid versus myeloid progenitors from purified cord blood precursor cells. Blood 8:3252–3258

McAdams TA, Miller WM, Papoutsakis ET (1996) Hematopoietic cell culture therapies (Part I): cell culture considerations. Trends Biotechnol 14:341–349

McAdams TA, Miller WM, Papoutsakis ET (1997) Variations in culture pH affect the cloning efficiency and differentiation of progenitor cells in ex vivo haemopoiesis. Brit J Haematol 97:889–895

Neildez-Nguyen TMA, Marden V, Wajcman H, et al. (2002) Human erythroid cells produced ex vivo at large scale differentiate into red blood cells in vivo. Nat Biotechnol 20:467–472

Patel VP, Lodish HF (1986) The fibronectin receptor on mammalian erythroid precursor cells: characterization and developmental regulation. J Cell Biol 102:449–456

Patel VP, Lodish HF (1987) A fibronectin matrix is required for differentiation of murine erythroleukemia cells into reticulocytes. J Cell Biol 105:3105–3118

Rosemblatt M, Vuillet-Gaugler MH, Leroy C, Coulombel L (1991) Coexpression of two fibronectin receptors, VLA-4 and VLA-5, by immature human erythroblastic precursor cells. J Clin Invest 87:6–11

Zermati Y, Varet B, Hermine O (2000a) TGF-beta1 drives and accelerates erythroid differentiation in the epo-dependent UT-7 cell line even in the absence of erythropoietin. Exp Hematol 28:256–266

Zermati Y, Fichelson S, Valensi F, Freyssinier JM, Rouyer-Fessard P, Cramer E, et al. (2000b) Transforming growth factor inhibits erythropoiesis by blocking proliferation and accelerating differentiation of erythroid progenitors. Exp Hematol 28:885–894

8 T-Cell Therapies
for EBV-Associated Malignancies

M. K. Brenner, C. Bollard, M. H. Huls, S. Gottschalk,
H. E. Heslop, C. M. Rooney

8.1 Introduction

Epstein-Barr virus (EBV) is associated with a range of malignant pathologies, each of which has a characteristic pattern of expression of viral latency genes (Heslop et al. 1996; Rooney et al. 1995, 1998). In Type 3 latency, essentially all viral latency proteins are expressed and the infected cells are highly immunogenic. This type of tumor therefore only occurs in immunocompromised patients (for example, after stem cell transplantation) and is associated with diffuse lymphoproliferative disease and immunoblastic B-cell lymphoma. In Type 2 latency, the less immunogenic EBV latency proteins are present [such as latent membrane protein of EBV (LMP)1 and LMP2, and EBNA1] and tumors with this latency pattern (e.g., Hodgkin's disease and nasopharyngeal carcinoma) may be found in immunocompetent patients. Type 1 latency produces the least immu-

nogenic tumors (e.g., Burkitt lymphoma) expressing EBNA1 protein
and BARFO transcripts. This article summarizes our experience over
the past 8 years in developing T-cell therapies to prevent and treat
EBV malignancies associated with viral latency Types 3 and 2.

8.2 Type 3 Latency:
Posttransplant Lymphoproliferative Disease

Epstein-Barr virus is a frequent cause of morbidity and mortality
after transplantation. The frequency of the complication depends on
the type of transplant and the degree of host immunosuppression,
but in transplants of the small bowel or stem cell transplants of T-
lymphocyte-depleted unrelated donor marrow, 20% or more of patients may be afflicted. EBV-associated problems after transplantation are due to uncontrolled proliferation of B cells with a Type 3 latency EBV gene expression. Because highly immunogenic viral latency proteins are present, the infected B cells are only able to survive and proliferate because of the patient's profound immunodeficiency. The disease may present acutely with fever, lymphadenopa-
thy (superficial or visceral), hepatosplenomegaly, and hemorrhage
from the gut or bladder due to erosion of infiltrating submucosal tumor. Occasionally the presentation is more insidious, occurring
many months or even years after the transplant itself. Diagnosis is
made from history and clinical and imaging evidence of lymphade-
nopathy and hepatosplenomegaly, a high LDH and – most specifically – from detection of a high level of EBV DNA in circulating cells
or present in plasma. Recently, anti-CD20 MAb (Rituximab) has
been shown to be effective in treating this disease, but resistant tumors are observed and the disease may recur.

An alternative treatment approach is to use virus-specific cytotoxic T lymphocyte (CTL) infusions. These are prepared from the
stem cell donor or from the solid organ transplant recipient by culturing T lymphocytes with donor/patient B-lymphocytes that have
been transformed into lymphoblastoid cell lines (LCL) by exposure
to a laboratory strain of Epstein-Barr virus. These LCL express the
same pattern of antigens as the tumor in the patients, allowing CTL
to be developed after 4–6 weeks of culture. The CTL are capable of

specifically recognizing the target antigens on the EBV-positive tumor cells. Importantly, it is possible to generate these EBV-specific T-cell lines even from patients who are receiving immunosuppressive agents including tacrolimus and Cyclosporin A (CSA). In more than 300 patients, we have established such lines with >98% success and similar results are now being obtained in other centers nationally and internationally. It is also possible to obtain EBV-specific T-cell lines from pediatric patients who are themselves EBV-negative, although this requires an extra selection step. This is a useful advance, since EBV-negative children receiving organs from EBV-positive donors have a high risk of developing EBV lymphoproliferation. Finally, we can genetically mark a small proportion of the CTL before infusion so that we can track them and determine their performance and fate in vivo (Heslop et al. 1996; Rooney et al. 1995, 1998).

These EBV-specific CTL have now successfully been given to patients after stem cell and solid organ transplantation. Their behavior is somewhat different in each group of patients. Following stem cell transplantation, infusion of as few as 10^7 CTL/m^2 is followed by a rapid in vivo expansion of virus-specific cells and an equally rapid return of raised EBV DNA levels to normal, in the 20% of patients who had viral DNA levels indicative of potential posttransplant lymphoproliferative disease (PTLD). None of 57 patients who received CTL as prophylaxis developed PTLD compared with 12% of controls. CTL also produced complete remissions in three patients with early PTLD and in two of three patients with bulky disease, all of whom received CTL as treatment. After solid organ transplantation, expansion in vivo is more gradual – perhaps because of the continued administration of immunosuppressive drugs, or because of the less "proliferative" environment. Nonetheless, after 2–3 injections of cells, a progressive rise in EBV-specific CTL can be measured by tetramer analysis, and this is associated with progressive control of EBV disease. Adverse events have proved minor, and have been limited to inflammatory changes at the sites of disease, in liver and lungs.

8.3 Type 2 Latency: Hodgkin's Disease

The malignant cells from 40% of cases of Hodgkin's disease also carry EBV and are potential targets for EBV-specific CTL. Unlike PTLD, which occurs only in patients with severe immune dysfunction, Hodgkin tumors develop and grow in patients who have a functional immune response to EBV. This capability is explained by the potent immune evasion strategies displayed by Hodgkin Reed-Sternberg (H-RS) cells (Poppema et al. 1995). They do not produce the immunodominant EBV proteins that make PTLD tumor cells highly immunogenic, expressing only four of the nine EBV latency proteins, LMP1, LMP2, EBNA1, and BARFO (Levitskaya et al. 1995; Herbst et al. 1991; Rickinson 1994). They also secrete cytokines and chemokines such as transforming growth factor (TGF)-β, IL-10, TARC, and IL-13 that inactivate professional antigen-presenting cells (APC), directly inhibit T cells and create a Th2 environment, which favors antibody production and inhibits Th1 CTL (Poppema et al. 1995; Hsu et al. 1993).

To determine whether "conventional" EBV-CTL are effective in Hodgkin's disease, 13 patients with EBV-positive HD received LCL-activated, gene-marked, EBV-specific CTL on two phase 1 dose escalation studies (Roskrow et al. 1998; Heslop et al. 2000; Smith et al. 1995). The studies were designed to enroll 3–6 patients on each of three dose levels of 4×10^6 CTL per m^2, 1.2×10^8 CTL per m^2, and 3×10^8 CTL per m^2. Eight patients received CTL as therapy for active disease after second or third relapse; six patients on dose level one, and two on dose level two. Five patients received CTL as adjuvant therapy after autologous stem cell rescue; three on dose level one, and two on level two. All blood was obtained with informed consent on locally and/or federally approved protocols.

The CTL used were genetically marked using a retrovirus vector containing the marker gene, *neo*, which allows us to determine the persistence and fate of the infused CTL.

EBV-specific CTL lines reactivated and expanded using the autologous LCL as APC, could be established from all patients, including those with bulky relapsed disease. CTL that could recognize EBV antigens actually present on HD cells (such as LMP1 and LMP2) were present, albeit with low frequency (<5%), in four of five EBV-specific CTL lines examined.

Immunological monitoring using a limiting dilution culture assay, and later Elispot and tetramer analysis, showed that the frequency of EBV-specific CTL increased by about one log, by 4 weeks after infusion, as measured in culture assays, while analysis of the frequency of LMP2a peptide tetramer-specific CTL increased up to 100-fold (Roskrow et al. 1998). Virus load, as measured by either standard or real time PCR was high in only one patient, but became undetectable in this patient and was reduced in most patients in whom virus load was detectable (Roskrow et al. 1998). This finding was important, since the only virus gene thought to be expressed in virus-infected, circulating normal B cells is thought to be LMP2, indicating that an LMP2-specific component was functional in vivo.

In situ marker gene-analysis demonstrated gene-marked CTL in a mediastinal tumor in one patient and in a malignant pleural effusion in a second patient, showing that CTL could home to sites of malignancy, despite the Th2 tumor environment (Roskrow et al. 1998; Gottschalk et al. 2002). Further, the marker gene could be detected for up to 10 months in patient peripheral blood using real time PCR amplification. Clinically, CTL produced resolution of B symptoms in three of four patients. Of eight patients who received CTL as therapy, one patient developed progressive disease and received only one infusion, one patient died of tumor erosion through a pulmonary artery 2 months after infusion, and five patients with relapsed disease had mixed tumor responses and survived 10–15 months after CTL infusion. The eighth patient survived for 18 months with stable disease and then had an allogeneic stem cell transplant with donor-derived CTL. He remains alive and well. Four of five patients who received CTL as adjuvant therapy post-SCT are alive and well 8 months to 2 years after CTL infusion. The fifth patient died of progressive disease, 3 months after CTL infusion.

8.4 Improving the Efficacy of Infused CTL

We are following a number of strategies to improve these outcomes. First we are continuing to dose escalate the number of CTL we give, although it is unlikely that this approach alone will prove beneficial. More productively, we are increasing the frequency of tumor reactive (i.e., LMP1 or LMP2 antigen-specific) T cells within the CTL lines. Recombinant adenovectors can express transgenic LMP2 in dendritic cells (DC), and transduced DC mature normally in response to maturation factors. When used to stimulate autologous peripheral blood mononuclear cells (PBMC) from patients and normal individuals, Ad-LMP2a-transduced DC reactivate LMP2-specific CTL, even from individuals who did not respond to LMP2 presented by the autologous LCL (Gahn et al. 2001). These CTL kill target cells expressing transgenic LMP2 from a vaccinia virus vector as well as LCL, which naturally express LMP2. A clinical protocol to use LMP2-specific CTL for the treatment of relapsed Hodgkin's disease has now been initiated.

Even LMP2-specific CTL may be unable to function optimally in the Hodgkin tumor environment of inhibitory cytokines. Therefore, we are also generating CTL that are genetically resistant to tumor-derived inhibition. The most potently inhibitory cytokine secreted by H-RS cells is TGF-β. When cultured in the presence of TGF-β, EBV-specific CTL failed to proliferate, failed to secrete cytokines such as GM-CSF and γ-IFN, and downregulated perforin, resulting in loss of cytotoxic activity (Bollard et al. 2002). Expression of a transgenic dominant-negative TGF-β receptor (Wieser et al. 1993) in CTL by transduction with a recombinant retrovirus vector rendered CTL resistant to the negative effects of TGF-β (Bollard et al. 2002). Thus transduced CTL continued to grow, to secrete GM-CSF and γ-IFN in response to antigenic stimulation, and killed EBV-infected target cells in the presence of concentrations of TGF-β that were inhibitory to vector-transduced CTL. These genetically modified CTL will require prolonged testing in animal models, since it is possible that loss of homeostatic pathways or overexpression of cytokines may allow uncontrolled proliferation of transduced T cells. We think this unlikely, because CTL are subject to multiple homeostatic pathways, such as Fas and Trail apoptotic pathways, as well as their dependence on the presence of antigen and growth factors (Lenardo et al. 1999). If our murine model continues to demonstrate the safety of TGF-β-resistant CTL, we will progress to clinical trials.

A second strategy of H-RS cells is to recruit Th2 cells, which can be seen surrounding each tumor cell like a bodyguard and creating a cytokine environment hostile to Th1 CTL (Skinnider and Mak

2002). IL-12 is a critical Th1 cytokine that determines the Th-type of the immune response and that has potent antitumor activity. We have transduced CTL lines with a fusion protein composed of the α and β chains of IL-12 connected by a flexible linker (Anderson et al. 1997). Functional IL-12 is secreted at levels several logs higher than from untransduced CTL, resulting in an increase in the expression of Th1 cytokines and a decrease in the expression of Th2 cytokines). IL-12, specifically targeted to tumor tissues using CTL, may overcome the dose-limiting toxicity of systemic recombinant human IL-12 used in clinical trials (Leonard et al. 1997). Intratumoral IL-12 may have several lines of antitumor activity. First, CTL expressing IL-12 may be resistant to the Th2 environment, second, IL-12 has potent direct antitumor effects, and third, IL-12 may break down the protective Th2 environment and destroy the tumor, even without direct cytolysis (Voest et al. 1995; Lucey et al. 1996).

8.5 Type 2 Latency: Nasopharyngeal Carcinoma

Nasopharyngeal carcinoma (NPC) is an epithelial tumor, and many patients with advanced stage disease fail to respond to conventional treatment. Even in the responders, relapse occurs in approximately 40%, and the standard treatment modalities of radiotherapy and chemotherapy are accompanied by severe long-term side effects including secondary malignancies. Since virtually all undifferentiated NPC are associated with Type 2 latency EBV, this type of tumor is an attractive candidate for immunotherapy targeted against tumor-associated EBV antigens. We have been successful in generating autologous EBV-specific CTL lines for NPC patients using our standardized method. As in Hodgkin's disease, previous exposure of NPC patients to radio- and chemotherapy does not prevent patient CTL lines expanding at similar rates as compared to those of healthy donors, indicating the feasibility of this approach. Adoptive transfer of EBV-specific CTLs has proven safe in all ten NPC patients treated. In six patients with refractory or relapsed disease, CTL infusion resulted in three complete response, one partial response, and stabilization of disease for >6 months in two cases. These results are promising and indicate the potential antitumor activity of EBV-specific CTLs in this patient group, but also suggest that, as in Hodgkin's disease, the T cells will need to be better targeted and made resistant to immune evasion strategies, possibilities we are now assessing.

8.6 Conclusion

At present, CTL are being used only in patients with advanced relapsed malignancies. As their safety and efficacy becomes better established we may expect their introduction earlier in the course of therapy where they may reduce the short- and long-term toxicities of standard radio- and chemotherapies. Further understanding of the ways in which immune evasion strategies can be counteracted in Hodgkin's disease may also be applied to the many other human tumors that are potentially immunogenic and use similar immune evasion strategies.

Acknowledgements. This work was supported by grants 1 RO1 CA74126 and 5M01RR000188-37 (GCRC) from the NIH and from the Department of Pediatrics, Baylor College of Medicine. HEH is the holder of a Distinguished Clinical Scientist award from the Doris Duke Foundation, CMB was supported by Gillson Longenbau Foundation, SG is a recipient of a Doris Duke Clinical Scientist Award.

References

Anderson R, Macdonald I, Corbett T, Hacking G, Lowdell MW, Prentice HG (1997) Construction and biological characterization of an interleukin-12 fusion protein (Flexi-12): delivery to acute myeloid leukemic blasts using adeno-associated virus. Hum Gene Ther 8:1125–1135

Bollard CM, Rossig C, Calonge MJ, et al. (2002) Adapting a transforming growth factor beta-related tumor protection strategy to enhance antitumor immunity. Blood 99:3179–3187

Gahn B, Siller-Lopez F, Pirooz AD, et al. (2001) Adenoviral gene transfer into dendritic cells efficiently amplifies the immune response to the LMP2A-antigen: a potential treatment strategy for Epstein-Barr virus-positive Hodgkin's lymphoma. Int J Cancer 93:706–713

Gottschalk S, Heslop HE, Rooney CM (2002) Treatment of Epstein-Barr virus-associated malignancies with specific T cells. Adv Cancer Res 84:175–201

Herbst H, Dallenback F, Hummel M, et al. (1991) Epstein-Barr virus latent membrane protein expression in Hodgkin and Reed-Sternberg cells. Proc Natl Acad Sci 88:4766–4770

Heslop H, Rooney C, Brenner M, et al. (2000) Administration of neomycin resistance gene-marked EBV-specific cytotoxic T-lymphocytes as therapy for patients receiving a bone marrow transplant for relapsed EBV-positive Hodgkin's disease. Hum Gene Ther 11:1465–1475

Heslop HE, Ng CYC, Li C, et al. (1996) Long-term restoration of immunity against Epstein-Barr virus infection by adoptive transfer of gene-modified virus-specific T lymphocytes. Nat Med 2:551–555

Hsu SM, Lin J, Xie SS, Hsu PL, Rich S (1993) Abundant expression of transforming growth factor-beta 1 and -beta 2 by Hodgkin's Reed-Sternberg cells and by reactive T lymphocytes in Hodgkin's disease. Hum Pathol 24:249–255

Lenardo M, Chan KM, Hornung F, et al. (1999) Mature T lymphocyte apoptosis-immune regulation in a dynamic and unpredictable antigenic environment. Annu Rev Immunol 17:221–253

Leonard JP, Sherman ML, Fisher GL, Buchanan LJ, Larsen G, Atkins MB, Sosman JA, Dutcher JP, Vogelzang NJ, Ryan JL (1997) Effects of single-dose interleukin-12 exposure on interleukin-12-associated toxicity and interferon-gamma production. Blood 90(7):2541–2548

Levitskaya J, Coram M, Levitsky V, et al. (1995) Inhibition of antigen processing by the internal repeat region of the Epstein-Barr virus nuclear antigen-1. Nature 375:685–688

Lucey DR, Clerici M, Shearer GM (1996) Type 1 and type 2 cytokine dysregulation in human infectious, neoplastic, and inflammatory diseases. Clin Microbiol Rev 9(4):532–562

Poppema S, Potters M, Visser L, van den Berg AM (1998) Immune escape mechanisms in Hodgkin's disease. Ann Oncol 9 (Suppl 5):S21–S24

Rickinson AB (1994) EBV infection and EBV-associated tumors. In: Minson AC, Neil JC, McRae MA (eds) Viruses and cancer. Cambridge University Press, Cambridge, pp 81–100

Rooney CM, Smith CA, Ng CYC, et al. (1995) Use of gene-modified virus-specific T lymphocytes to control Epstein-Barr virus-related lymphoproliferation. Lancet 345:9–13

Rooney CM, Smith CA, Ng CYC, et al. (1998) Infusion of cytotoxic T cells for the prevention and treatment of Epstein-Barr virus-induced lymphoma in allogeneic transplant recipients. Blood 92:1549–1555

Roskrow MA, Rooney CM, Heslop HE, et al. (1998a) Administration of neomycin resistance gene marked EBV-specific cytotoxic T-lymphocytes to patients with relapsed EBV-positive Hodgkin's disease. Hum Gene Ther 9:1237–1250

Roskrow MA, Suzuki N, Gan Y-J, et al. (1998b) EBV-specific cytotoxic T lymphocytes for the treatment of patients with EBV positive relapsed Hodgkin's disease. Blood 91:2925–2934

Skinnider BF, Mak TW (2002) The role of cytokines in classical Hodgkin lymphoma. Blood 99:4283–4297

Smith CA, Ng CYC, Heslop HE, et al. (1995) Production of genetically modified EBV-specific cytotoxic T cells for adoptive transfer to patients at high risk of EBV-associated lymphoproliferative disease. J Hematother 4:73–79

Voest EE, Kenyon BM, O'Reilly MS, Truitt G, D'Amato RJ, Folkman J (1995) Inhibition of angiogenesis in vivo by interleukin 12. J Natl Cancer Inst 87(8):581–586

Wieser R, Attisano L, Wrana JL, Massague J (1993) Signaling activity of transforming growth factor beta type II receptors lacking specific domains in the cytoplasmic region. Mol Cell Biol 13:7239–7247

9 Peptide Vaccination of Myeloid Leukemia

D. Kurbegov, J. J. Molldrem

9.1 Introduction

The most compelling evidence that lymphocytes mediate an antitumor effect comes from studies where allogeneic donor lymphocyte infusions (DLI) have been used to treat relapse of myeloid leukemia after allogeneic BMT (Giralt and Kolb 1996; Kolb and Holler 1997; Kolb et al. 1995, 1996; Antin 1993). Lymphocyte transfusion from the original bone marrow (BM) donor induces both hematological and cytogenetic responses in approximately 70%–80% of patients with CML in chronic phase (CP) (Kolb et al. 1996). A complete cytogenetic response is usually obtained between 1 and 4 months after DLI (van Rhee et al. 1994), and approximately 80% of responders will achieve reverse transcriptase-polymerase chain reaction (RTPCR) negativity for the bcr-abl translocation [the fusion product of the t(9;22) translocation found in CML] within a mean of 6 months (van Rhee et al. 1994). Acute myelogenous leukemia (AML) is also susceptible to the graft-versus-leukemia (GVL) effect, with 15%–40% of patients obtaining remission with DLI alone (Collins et al. 1997). While signifi-

cant graft-versus-host disease (GVHD) occurs in 50% of patients
treated with DLI, and disease response occurs in 90% of CML patients, 55% of patients who do not experience GVHD also have disease response (Giralt and Kolb 1996; Kolb and Holler 1997). This
demonstrates that GVL is separable from GVHD in some patients,
and several potential antigens that drive the donor's lymphocyte response preferentially against the leukemia have been identified. There
is also evidence of an autologous immune response against both CML
and AML, which is directed against some of the same antigens. Remissions after DLI for AML are generally not as durable as those obtained
in chronic phase CML, which may reflect the rapid kinetics of tumor
growth outpacing the kinetics of the developing immune response as
well as a potentially less immunogenic target cell. However, if more
antigens could be determined, and if large numbers of antigen-specific cytotoxic T lymphocytes (CTLs) could be elicited via vaccination
strategies, it would allow for development of leukemia-specific therapies.

To understand the nature of vaccine-induced T cell immunity, we
will first review some of the principles of antigen recognition and
highlight a recent discovery that has aided our ability to study T cell
interactions. T cells recognize peptide antigens that are presented on
the cell surface in combination with major histocompatibility complex (MHC) antigens. Peptides derived from cytoplasmic proteins
that are 8–11 amino acids in length bind in the groove of class I
MHC molecules and are transported via the endoplasmic reticulum
to the cell surface. Larger peptides, typically 12–18 amino acids in
length, that are derived from the processing of extracellular proteins,
bind class II MHC molecules and are presented to T cells on the
cell surface. Both peptide/MHC-I and peptide/MHC-II are recognized by the heterodimeric T cell receptor (TCR) and CD8 or CD4
T lymphocytes, respectively, with weak affinity and rapid off rates.
Points of contact between the TCR and the peptide/MHC surface include surface amino acids contributed by the two α-helical domains
of the MHC molecule that flank the peptide antigen binding pocket
as well as amino acids from the peptide itself.

Our understanding of the nature of antigen-specific T cell responses has been greatly improved by the discovery that antigen-specific TCR can be reversibly labeled with soluble peptide/MHC tetra-

mers (Altman et al. 1996). Peptide antigen, $\beta 2$ microglobulin and the MHC-I heavy chain are folded together and, via a biotinylation signal sequence at the C-terminus of the MHC-I heavy chain, are linked covalently to streptavidin in a 4:1 molecular ratio. When the streptavidin molecule is linked to a fluorescent dye such as phyco-erythrin, the resulting peptide/MHC tetramers can be used to identify antigen-specific T cells by FACS analysis because of their higher binding avidity to the cognate TCR. Using tetramers, it has been determined that up to 45% of all peripheral circulating T cells may be specific for a single dominant antigen at the height of an immune response to EBV infection (Callan et al. 1998) and similar dominance may be seen during other viral infections (Komanduri et al. 1998, 2001). Tetramers have also been used to study immune responses to tumor antigens (Lee et al. 1999), and they have also aided in their discovery (Molldrem et al. 2000).

9.2 Potential Target Antigens

Various methods have been used to determine the nature of the target antigens involved in leukemia immunity. For instance, tissue-restricted minor histocompatibility antigens (mHA) that are derived from proteins expressed only in hematopoietic tissue have been shown to be the targets of alloreactive T cells (Murata et al. 2003; den Haan et al. 1995, 1998; Warren et al. 1998; Dolstra et al. 1997). These mHA often result from polymorphic differences between donor and recipient in the coding regions of peptide antigens that bind within the groove of MHC molecules and are recognized by donor T cells. Recently, however, a newly described mHA was found to result from differential expression in donor and recipient due to a gene deletion (Murata et al. 2003). Heterologous T cell clones that demonstrate alloreactivity toward mHA have been established from patients with severe GVHD following BMT with an HLA-matched donor (Faber et al. 1995 a, b, 1996; van der Harst et al. 1994). Some of these mHA-specific CTL clones react only with hematopoietic-derived cells, suggesting tissue specificity (Faber et al. 1996), and therefore potentially shared antigens on leukemia. In one study, GVHD correlated closely with differences in the minor antigen

HA-1 in HLA-identical sibling transplants (Goulmy et al. 1996). Expression of two human mHAs, identified as HA-1 and HA-2, is confined to hematopoietic tissues, and HA-2 was identified as a peptide derived from the nonfilament-forming class I myosin family by using mHA-reactive CTL clones to screen peptide fractions eluted from MHC class I molecules (den Haan et al. 1995). While this methodology has successfully defined the first CTL alloantigens, it is labor intensive and it is unclear whether CTL specific for any minor antigens identified thus far convey only leukemia-specific immunity without concomitant GVHD. Immunization of leukemia patients after allogeneic stem cell transplant (vaccination by proxy) with mHA may promote GVL and reduce GVHD if appropriate hematopoietic-restricted mHA could be targeted (such as HA-1 or HA-2). In a recent report of 3 CML patients that received DLI after relapse, however, GVHD occurred in each patient concomitant to a rise in HA-1- or HA-2-specific CTL and cytogenetic remission, albeit grade 2 or less (Marijt et al. 2003). Perhaps more importantly, a practical limit of immunotherapy targeting these mHAs is that only 10% of individuals would be expected to have the relevant HA-1 alternate allele, and less than 1% would have the HA-2 alternate allele, which makes donor availability quite limiting.

An alternative immunological method to determine leukemia-specific CTL epitopes has been applied to determine whether BCR-ABL fusion region peptides could be used to elicit CML-specific T cell responses. Using this method, peptides are synthesized based upon an "educated guess" strategy about which proteins are potential target antigens for a selective antileukemia CTL response. The proteins are then examined for short peptides that fit the binding motif of the most common HLA alleles. These peptides are then synthesized, HLA binding is confirmed, and peptide-specific CTL responses are elicited in vitro. Since BCR-ABL is present in nearly all Philadelphia chromosome-positive CML patients, it is thought to represent a potentially unique leukemia antigen. The ABL coding sequences upstream (5′) of exon II and chromosome 9 are translocated to chromosome 22 and fused in-frame with the BCR gene downstream (3′) of exon III, resulting in the most common chimeric mRNA transcript (b3a2), which is translated into a chimeric protein ($p210^{BCR-ABL}$). Translation of b3a2 mRNA results in the coding of a unique amino acid (lysine) within the fusion region. Some HLA-A2, -A3, -A22, and B8-restricted overlapping peptides inclusive of this lysine could bind to their respective HLA alleles and could be used to elicit T cell proliferative responses when the peptide was either pulsed onto HLA-matched normal antigen presenting cells or onto HLA-B8 positive CML cells (Dermime et al. 1995; Bocchia et al. 1995, 1996). However, when the b3a2 peptides were used to elicit b3a2-specific T lymphocyte lines in vitro, the resulting T cells could not specifically lyse fresh CML cells which had not previously been pulsed with the peptide (Bocchia et al. 1996). This could be due to a low affinity of the peptide-specific CTL or the peptide may not be processed or presented in CML cells. More recently, however, b3a2-specific CTL were identified in the peripheral blood of chronic-phase CML patients using soluble b3a2 peptide/MHC tetramers (Clark et al. 2001). Although the tetramer-positive CTL from the patients were not examined for their ability to kill autologous CML target cells, b3a2-specific CTL elicited in vitro from healthy donors were able to kill CML cells. This suggests that bcr-abl fusion peptides may also be targets of CTL immunity.

To adapt what has been learned about immunity against solid tumor antigens to the study of myeloid leukemia antigens, we studied myeloid-restricted proteins that are highly expressed in the leukemia relative to normal hematopoietic progenitors. Myeloid leukemias express a number of differentiation antigens associated with granule formation. An example of an aberrantly expressed tumor antigen in human leukemia is proteinase 3 (Pr3), a 26 kDa neutral serine protease that is stored in primary azurophil granules and is maximally expressed at the promyelocyte stage of myeloid differentiation (Sturrock et al. 1992; Chen et al. 1994; Muller-Berat et al. 1994). Pr3 and two other azurophil granule proteins, neutrophil elastase and azurocidin, are coordinately regulated and the transcription factors PU.1 and C/EBPa, which are responsible for normal myeloid differentiation from stem cells to monocytes or granulocytes, are important in mediating their expression (Zhang et al. 2002). These transcription factors have been implicated in leukemogenesis (Behre et al. 1999), and Pr3 itself may also be important in maintaining a leukemia phenotype since Pr3 antisense oligonucleotides halt cell division and induce maturation of the HL-60 promyelocytic leukemia cell line (Bories et al. 1989).

We have also studied another myeloid-restricted protein, myelo-peroxidase (MPO), a heme protein synthesized during very early myeloid differentiation that constitutes the major component of neutrophil azurophilic granules. Produced as a single chain precursor, myeloperoxidase is subsequently cleaved into a light and heavy chain. The mature myeloperoxidase enzyme is composed of two light chains and two heavy chains (Borregaard and Cowland 1997) that produce hypohalous acids central to the microbicidal activity of neutrophils. Importantly, MPO and Pr3 are both overexpressed in a variety of myeloid leukemia cells including 75% of CML patients, approximately 50% of acute myeloid leukemia patients, and approximately 30% of myelodysplastic syndrome patients (Dengler et al. 1995).

What may be critical for our ability to identify T cell antigens in these proteins is the observation that Pr3 is the target of autoimmune attack in Wegener's granulomatosis (Franssen et al. 1996) and MPO is a target antigen in patients with small vessel vasculitis (Borregaard and Cowland 1997; Brouwer et al. 1994; Franssen et al. 2000). There is evidence for both T cell and humoral immunity in patients with these diseases. Wegener's granulomatosis is associated with production of *cytoplasmic* antineutrophil cytoplasmic antibodies (cANCA) with specificity for Pr3 (Williams et al. 1994), while microscopic polyangiitis and ChurgStrauss syndrome are associated with the production of *perinuclear* ANCA (pANCA) antibodies with specificity for MPO (Jennette et al. 2001; Savige et al. 1999). T cells taken from affected individuals proliferate in response to crude extracts from neutrophil granules and to the purified proteins (Brouwer et al. 1994; Ballieux et al. 1995). These findings suggest that T cell responses against these proteins might be relatively easy to elicit in vitro using a deductive strategy to identify HLA-restricted peptide epitopes. Based on this hypothesis, we identified PR1, an HLA-A2.1-restricted nonamer derived from Pr3, as a leukemia-associated antigen (Molldrem et al. 1996, 1997, 1999, 2000) by first searching the length of the protein using the HLA-A2.1 binding motif, the most prevalent HLA allele. Peptides predicted to have high affinity binding to HLA-A2.1 were synthesized, confirmed to bind, and then used to elicit peptide-specific cytotoxic T lymphocytes (CTL) in vitro from healthy donor lymphocytes.

We have found that PR1 can be used to elicit CTL from HLA-A2.1[+] normal donors in vitro, and that T cell immunity to PR1 is present in healthy donors and in many patients with CML that are in remission. These PR1-specific CTL show preferential cytotoxicity toward allogeneic HLA-A2.1[+] myeloid leukemia cells over HLA-identical normal donor marrow (Molldrem et al. 1996). In addition, PR1-specific CTL inhibit colony-forming unit granulocyte-macrophage (CFU-GM) from the marrow of CML patients, but not CFU-GM from normal HLA-matched donors (Molldrem et al. 1997), suggesting that leukemia progenitors are also targeted.

Using PR1/HLA-A2 tetramers to detect CTL specific for PR1 (PR1-CTL), we found a significant correlation with cytogenetic remission after treatment with interferon-α and the presence of PR1-CTL (Molldrem et al. 2000). Somewhat surprisingly, PR1-CTL were also identified in the peripheral blood of some allogeneic transplant recipients who achieved molecular remission and who had converted to 100% donor chimerism. PR1/HLA-A2 tetramer-sorted allogeneic CTL from patients in remission were able to kill CML cells but not normal bone marrow cells in 4-h cytotoxicity assays, thus demonstrating that the PR1 self-antigen is also recognized by allogeneic CTL (Molldrem et al. 2000). These studies have established PR1 as a human leukemia-associated antigen and they established that PR1-specific CTL contribute to the elimination of CML (Molldrem et al. 2000).

Recently, we found another peptide, referred to as MY4, a 9 amino acid peptide derived from MPO that binds to HLA-A2.1, can be used to elicit CTL from HLA-A2.1[+] normal donors in vitro (Braunschweig et al. 2000). MY4-specific CTL show preferential cytotoxicity toward allogeneic HLA-A2.1[+] myeloid leukemia cells over HLA-identical normal donor marrow (Braunschweig et al. 2000). MY4-specific CTL also inhibit CFU-GM from the marrow of CML patients, but not CFU-GM from normal HLA-matched donors. Like PR1, MY4 is therefore a peptide antigen that can elicit leukemia-specific CTL.

Several other HLA-restricted epitopes have been identified as potentially relevant leukemia-associated antigens. The Wilm's tumor antigen-1 (WT1) has emerged as a very potent immunogen containing multiple unique HLA-restricted epitopes (Azuma et al. 2002; Bellantuono et al. 2002; Gao et al. 2000; Scheibenbogen et al. 2002;

Oka et al. 2000), and it may also be a marker of minimal residual disease since it is aberrantly expressed in both myeloid and lymphoid acute leukemia (Bergmann et al. 1997a,b; Brieger et al. 1995). Various surface molecules on leukemia cells, such as CD45, present on all hematopoietic cells, and CD33 and CD19 on myeloid and lymphoid cells, respectively, have also been studied by deductive means to uncover potentially immunogenic epitopes (Chen et al. 1995; Raptis et al. 1998; Amrolia et al. 2002). While some HLA-restricted epitopes have been identified, it is unclear if any of these are leukemia-associated antigens. The method of serologic screening of cDNA expression libraries with autologous serum (SEREX) has also been used to identify MAGE-1 and to confirm WT1 as potential leukemia-associated antigens, although there may be some controversy whether the MAGE proteins are expressed in leukemia blasts (Chambost et al. 2001).

In addition to these tissue-restricted epitopes in myeloid leukemias, other potential antigens that might be useful as target antigens in vaccine therapies include the idiotypes associated with lymphoid malignancies, such as immunoglobulin idiotypes and the CDR3 variable region associated with the TCR. Furthermore, antigens that are aberrantly expressed in most tumors such as telomerase and CYP1B1 contain epitopes that are recognized by CTL in vitro, which preferentially kill tumor cells, but not normal cells. Other potential targets include antigens from virus-induced hematological malignancies, such as the EBV antigens.

9.3 Clinical Trial

The PR1 peptide is undergoing phase I/II study, and the single peptide epitope is combined with incomplete Freund's adjuvant and GM-CSF and administered every 3 weeks for a total of three total vaccinations. Patients with AML, CML, and MDS are eligible, and the first nine patients were reported at the annual American Society of Hematology meeting in 2002. To judge whether a clinical response was due to the vaccine, eligible patients were required to have progression, relapse, or ≥2nd CR (AML patients only) prior to vaccination. Immune responses, measured using PR1/HLA-A2 tetramers, were noted in five of the patients and clinical remissions were noted in four of these patients. Notably, the TCR avidity of the vaccine-induced PR1-specific CTL was higher in the clinical responders than in the nonresponders, and durable molecular remissions were noted in two refractory AML patients that were followed for 8 months to nearly 3 years.

9.4 Conclusion

In summary, we are beginning to learn more about the nature of the antigens targeted by T cells that mediate autologous antileukemia immunity and those that are the targets of the GVL effect. Some self-antigens might also be the targets of alloreactive CTL, as we have shown for PR1. If more antigens were identified, logical immunotherapy strategies such as vaccines or adoptive cellular therapies could be tested in patients. Obstacles to this approach remain, however. We must identify which of the hematopoietic tissue-restricted peptides are recognized by T cells and we must improve our understanding of the nature of peripheral T cell tolerance so that we might break immune tolerance to certain peptide determinants without causing potentially destructive autoimmunity. In the future, allogeneic stem cell transplantation is likely to evolve as a platform for delivering antigen-specific adoptive cellular therapies and for post-transplant vaccination strategies where donor CTL are elicited in the recipient. Both autologous and allogeneic transplant may reset T cell homeostasis and allow a more complete T cell repertoire to emerge postgrafting that could be further expanded selectively against tumor antigens by vaccination posttransplant, as in a vaccination by proxy therapy in the case of allogeneic transplantation.

References

Altman JD, Moss PA, Goulder PJ, Barouch DH, McHeyzer-Williams MG, Bell JI, McMichael AJ, Davis MM (1996) Phenotypic analysis of antigen-specific T lymphocytes. Science 274(5284):94–96

Amrolia PJ, Reid SD, Gao L, Schultheis B, Dotti G, Brenner MK, Melo JV, Goldman JM, Stauss HJ (2002) Allo-restricted cytotoxic t cells specific for human CD45 show potent antileukemic activity. Blood 101(3):1007–1014

Antin JH (1993) Graft-versus-leukemia: no longer an epiphenomenon. Blood 82:2273–2277

Azuma T, Makita M, Ninomiya K, Fujita S, Harada M, Yasukawa M (2002) Identification of a novel WT1-derived peptide which induces human leukocyte antigenA24-restricted anti-leukaemia cytotoxic T lymphocytes. Br J Haematol 116(3):601–603

Ballieux BE, van der Burg SH, Hagen EC, van der Woude FJ, Melief CJ, Daha MR (1995) Cell-mediated autoimmunity in patients with Wegener's granulomatosis (WG). Clin Exp Immunol 100(2):186–193

Behre G, Zhang P, Zhang DE, Tenen DG (1999) Analysis of the modulation of transcriptional activity in myelopoiesis and leukemogenesis. Methods 17(3):231–237

Bellantuono I, Gao L, Parry S, Marley S, Dazzi F, Apperley J, Goldman JM, Stauss HJ (2002) Two distinct HLAA0201-presented epitopes of the Wilms tumor antigen 1 can function as targets for leukemia-reactive CTL. Blood 100(10):3835–3837

Bergmann L, Maurer U, Weidmann E (1997a) Wilms tumor gene expression in acute myeloid leukemias. Leuk Lymphoma 25(5/6):435–443

Bergmann L, Miething C, Maurer U, Brieger J, Karakas T, Weidmann E, Hoelzer D (1997b) High levels of Wilms' tumor gene (wt1) mRNA in acute myeloid leukemias are associated with a worse long-term outcome. Blood 90(3):1217–1225

Bocchia M, Wentworth PA, Southwood S, Sidney J, McGraw K, Scheinberg DA, Sette A (1995) Specific binding of leukemia oncogene fusion protein peptides to HLA class I molecules. Blood 85(10):2680–2684

Bocchia M, Korontsvit T, Xu Q, Mackinnon S, Yang SY, Sette A, Scheinberg DA (1996) Specific human cellular immunity to bcr-abl oncogene-derived peptides. Blood 87(9):3587–3592

Bories D, Raynal MC, Solomon DH, Darzynkiewicz Z, Cayre YE (1989) Down-regulation of a serine protease, myeloblastin, causes growth arrest and differentiation of promyelocytic leukemia cells. Cell 59:959–968

Borregaard N, Cowland JB (1997) Granules of the human neutrophilic polymorphonuclear leukocyte. Blood 89(10):3503–3521

Braunschweig I, Wang C, Molldrem J (2000) Cytotoxic T lymphocytes (CTL) specific for myeloperoxidase-derived HLA-A2-restricted peptides specifically lyse AML and CML cells. Blood 96(11):3291

Brieger J, Weidmann E, Maurer U, Hoelzer D, Mitrou PS, Bergmann L (1995) The Wilms' tumor gene is frequently expressed in acute myeloblastic leukemias and may provide a marker for residual blast cells detectable by PCR. Ann Oncol 6(8):811–816

Brouwer E, Stegeman CA, Huitema MG, Limburg PC, Kallenberg CG (1994) T cell reactivity to proteinase 3 and myeloperoxidase in patients with Wegener's granulomatosis (WG). Clin Exp Immunol 98(3):448–453

Callan MF, Tan L, Annels N, Ogg GS, Wilson JD, O'Callaghan CA, Steven N, McMichael AJ, Rickinson AB (1998) Direct visualization of antigen-specific CD8[+] T cells during the primary immune response to Epstein-Barr virus in vivo. J Exp Med 87(9):1395–1402

Chambost H, van Baren N, Brasseur F, Olive D (2001) MAGE-A genes are not expressed in human leukemias. Leukemia 15(11):1769–1771

Chen T, Meier R, Ziemiecki A, Fey MF, Tobler A (1994) Myeloblastinproteinase 3 belongs to the set of negatively regulated primary response genes expressed during in vitro myeloid differentiation. Biochem Biophys Res Commun 200(2):1130–1135

Chen W, Chatta K, Rubin W, et al. (1995) Polymorphic segments of CD45 can serve as targets for GVHD and GVL responses (abstract). Blood 86:158a

Clark RE, Dodi IA, Hill SC, Lill JR, Aubert G, Macintyre AR, Rojas J, Bourdon A, Bonner PL, Wang L, Christmas SE, Travers PJ, Creaser CS, Rees RC, Madrigal JA (2001) Direct evidence that leukemic cells present HLA-associated immunogenic peptides derived from the BCR ABL b3a2 fusion protein. Blood 98(10):2887–2893

Collins RH Jr, Shpilberg O, Drobyski WR, Porter DL, Giralt S, Champlin R, Goodman SA, Wolff SN, Hu W, Verfaillie C, List A, Dalton W, Ognoskie N, Chetrit A, Antin JH, Nemunaitis J (1997) Donorleukocyte infusions in 140 patients with relapsed malignancy after allogeneic bone marrow transplantation. J Clin Oncol 5(2):433–444

den Haan JM, Sherman NE, Blokland E, Huczko E, Koning F, Drijfhout JW, Skipper J, Shabanowitz J, Hunt DF, Engelhard VH, et al. (1995) Identification of a graft versus host disease-associated human minor histocompatibility antigen. Science 268:1476–1480

den Haan JM, Meadows LM, Wang W, Pool J, Blokland E, Bishop TL, Reinhardus C, Shabanowitz J, Offringa R, Hunt DF, Engelhard VH, Goulmy E (1998) The minor histocompatibility antigen HA-1: a diallelic gene with a single amino acid polymorphism. Science 279:1054–1057

Dengler R, Munstermann U, al-Batran S, Hausner I, Faderl S, Nerl C, Emmerich B (1995) Immunocytochemical and flow cytometric detection of proteinase 3 (myeloblastin) in normal and leukaemic myeloid cells. Br J Haematol 89(2):250–257

Dermime S, Molldrem J, Parker KC, et al. (1995) Human CD8[+] T lymphocytes recognize the fusion region of bcrlabl hybrid protein present in chronic myelogenous leukemia (abstract). Blood 86:158a

Dolstra H, Fredrix H, Preijers F, Goulmy E, Figdor CG, de Witte TM, van de Wiel-van Kemenade E (1997) Recognition of a B cell leukemia-associated minor histocompatibility antigen by CTL. J Immunol 158(2):560–565

Faber LM, van der Hoeven J, Goulmy E, Hooftman-den Otter AL, van Luxemburg-Heijs SA, Willemze R, Falkenburg JH (1995a) Recognition of clonogenic leukemic cells, remission bone marrow and HLA-identical donor bone marrow by CD8[+] or CD4[+] minor histocompatibility antigen-specific cytotoxic T lymphocytes. J Clin Invest 96(2):877–883

Faber LM, van Luxemburg-Heijs SA, Veenhof WF, Willemze R, Falkenburg JH (1995b) Generation of CD4$^+$ cytotoxic T-lymphocyte clones from a patient with severe graft-versus-host disease after allogeneic bone marrow transplantation: implications for graft-versus-leukemia reactivity. Blood 86(7):2821–2828

Faber LM, van Luxemburg-Heijs SA, Rijnbeek M, Willemze R, Falkenburg JH (1996) Minor histocompatibility antigen-specific, leukemia-reactive cytotoxic T cell clones can be generated in vitro without in vivo priming using chronic myeloid leukemia cells as stimulators in the presence of alpha-interferon. Biol Blood Marrow Transplant 2(1):31–36

Franssen CF, Tervaert JW, Stegeman CA, Kallenberg CG (1996) c ANCA as a marker of Wegener's disease. Lancet 347(8994):116; discussion 118

Franssen CF, Stegeman CA, Kallenberg CG, Gans RO, De Jong PE, Hoorntje SJ, Tervaert JW (2000) Antiproteinase 3- and antimyeloperoxidase-associated vasculitis. Kidney Int 57(6):2195–2206

Gao L, Bellantuono I, Elsasser A, Marley SB, Gordon MY, Goldman JM, Stauss HJ (2000) Selective elimination of leukemic CD34($^+$) progenitor cells by cytotoxic T lymphocytes specific for WT1. Blood 95(7):2198–2203

Giralt SA, Kolb HJ (1996) Donor lymphocyte infusions. Curr Opin Oncol 8(2):96–102

Goulmy E, Schipper R, Pool J, Blokland E, Falkenburg JH, Vossen J, Gratwohl A, Vogelsang GB, van Houwelingen HC, van Rood JJ (1996) Mismatches of minor histocompatibility antigens between HLA-identical donors and recipients and the development of graft-versus-host disease alter bone marrow transplantation. N Engl J Med 334(5):281–285

Jennette JC, Thomas DB, Falk RJ (2001) Microscopic polyangiitis (microscopic polyarteritis). Semin Diagn Pathol 18(1):3–13

Kolb HJ, Holler E (1997) Adoptive immunotherapy with donor lymphocyte transfusions. Curr Opin Oncol 9(2):139–145

Kolb HJ, Schattenberg A, Goldman JM, et al. (1995) Graft-versus-leukemia effect of donor lymphocyte transfusions in marrow grafted patients. European Group for Blood and Marrow Transplantation Working Party Chronic Leukemia. Blood 86(5):2041–2050

Kolb HJ, Mittermuller J, Holler E, Thalmeier K, Bartram CR (1996) Graft-versus-host reaction spares normal stem cells in chronic myelogenous leukemia. Bone Marrow Transplant 17(3):449–452

Komanduri KV, Viswanathan MN, Wieder ED, Schmidt DK, Bredt BM, Jacobson MA, McCune JM (1998) Restoration of cytomegalovirus-specific CD4$^+$ T lymphocyte responses after ganciclovir and highly active antiretroviral therapy in individuals infected with HIV-1. Nat Med 4(8):953–956

Komanduri KV, Donahoe SM, Moretto WJ, Schmidt DK, Gillespie G, Ogg GS, Roederer M, Nixon DF, McCune JM (2001) Direct measurement of CD4$^+$ and CD8$^+$ T-cell responses to CMV in HIV-1-infected subjects. Virology 279(2):459–470

Lee PP, Yee C, Savage PA, Fong L, Brockstedt D, Weber JS, Johnson D, Swetter S, Thompson J, Greenberg PD, Roederer M, Davis MM (1999) Characterization of circulating T cells specific for tumor-associated antigens in melanoma patients. Nat Med 5(6):677

Marijt WA, Heemskerk MH, Kloosterboer FM, Goulmy E, Kester MG, van der Hoorn MA, van Luxemburg-Heys SA, Hoogeboom M, Mutis T, Drijfhout JW, van Rood JJ, Willemze R, Falkenburg JH (2003) Hematopoiesis-restricted minor histocompatibility antigens HA-1- or HA-2-specific T cells can induce complete remissions of relapsed leukemia. Proc Natl Acad Sci 100(5):2742–2747

Molldrem J, Dermime S, Parker K, Jiang YZ, Mavroudis D, Hensel N, Fukushima P, Barrett AJ (1996) Targeted T-cell therapy for human leukemia: cytotoxic T lymphocytes specific for a peptide derived from proteinase 3 preferentially lyse human myeloid leukemia cells. Blood 88(7):2450–2457

Molldrem JJ, Clave E, Jiang YZ, Mavroudis D, Raptis A, Hensel N, Agarwala V, Barrett AJ (1997) Cytotoxic T lymphocytes specific for a nonpolymorphic proteinase 3 peptide preferentially inhibit chronic myeloid leukemia colony-forming units. Blood 90(7):2529–2534

Molldrem JJ, Lee PP, Wang C, Champlin RE, Davis MM (1999) A PR1-human leukocyte antigen A2 tetramer can be used to isolate low-frequency cytotoxic T lymphocytes from healthy donors that selectively lyse chronic myelogenous leukemia. Cancer Res 59(11):2675–2681

Molldrem JJ, Lee PP, Wang C, Felio K, Kantarjian HM, Champlin RE, Davis MM (2000) Evidence that specific T lymphocytes may participate in the elimination of chronic myelogenous leukemia. Nat Med 6(9):1018–1023

Muller-Berat N, Minowada J, Tsuji-Takayama K, Drexler H, Lanotte M, Wieslander J, Wiik A (1994) The phylogeny of proteinase 3 myeloblastin, the autoantigen in Wegener's granulomatosis, and myeloperoxidase as shown by immunohistochemical studies in human leukemic cell lines. Clin Immunol Immunopathol 70(1):51–59

Murata M, Warren EH, Riddell ER (2003) A human minor histocompatibility antigen resulting from differential expression due to a gene deletion. J Exp Med 197(10):1279–1289

Oka Y, Elisseeva OA, Tsuboi A, Ogawa H, Tamaki H, Li H, Oji Y, Kim EH, Soma T, Asada M, Ueda K, Maruya E, Saji H, Kishimoto T, Udaka K, Sugiyama H (2000) Human cytotoxic T-lymphocyte responses specific for peptides of the wild-type Wilms' tumor gene (WT1) product. Immunogenetics 51(2):99–107

Raptis A, Clave E, Mavroudis D, Molldrem J, Van Rhee F, Barrett AJ (1998) Polymorphism in CD33 and CD34 genes: a source of minor histocompatibility antigens in haemopoietic progenitor cells? Br J Haematol 102(5):1354–1358

Savige J, Gillis D, Benson E, Davies D, Esnault V, Falk RJ, Hagen EC, Jayne D, Jennette JC, Paspaliaris B, Pollock W, Pusey C, Savage CO, Silvestrini R, van der Woude F, Wieslander J, Wiik A (1999) International Consensus Statement on Testing and Reporting of Antineutrophil Cytoplasmic Antibodies (ANCA). Am J Clin Pathol 111(4):507–513

Scheibenbogen C, Letsch A, Thiel E, Schmittel A, Mailaender V, Baerwolf S, Nagorsen D, Keilholz U (2002) CD8 T-cell responses to Wilms tumor gene product WT1 and proteinase 3 in patients with acute myeloid leukemia. Blood 100(6):2132–2137

Sturrock AB, Franklin KF, Rao G, Marshall BC, Rebentisch MB, Lemons RS, Hoidal JR (1992) Structure, chromosomal assignment, and expression of the gene for proteinase 3. J Biol Chem 267:21193–21199

van der Harst D, Goulmy E, Falkenburg JH, Kooij-Winkelaar YM, van Luxemburg-Heijs SA, Goselink HM, Brand A (1994) Recognition of minor histocompatibility antigens on lymphocytic and myeloid leukemic cells by cytotoxic T-cell clones. Blood 83(4):1060–1066

van Rhee F, Lin F, Cullis JO, Spencer A, Cross NC, Chase A, Garicochea B, Bungey J, Barrett J, Goldman JM (1994) Relapse of chronic myeloid leukemia after allogeneic bone marrow transplant: the case for giving donor lymphocyte transfusions before the onset of hematological relapse. Blood 83:3377–3383

Warren EH, Greenberg PD, Riddell SR (1998) Cytotoxic T-lymphocyte-defined human minor histocompatibility antigens with a restricted tissue distribution. Blood 91(6):2197–2207

Williams RC Jr, Staud R, Malone CC, Payabyab J, Byres L, Underwood D (1994) Epitopes an proteinase 3 recognized by antibodies from patients with Wegener's granulomatosis. J Immunol 152:4722–4732

Zhang P, Nelson E, Radomska HS, Iwasaki-Arai J, Akashi K, Friedman AD, Tenen DG (2002) Induction of granulocytic differentiation by 2 pathways. Blood 99(12):4406–4412

10 Hematopoietic Cell Transplantation after Nonmyeloablative Conditioning

M. L. Sorror, R. Storb

10.1 Introduction

Allogeneic hematopoietic cell transplantation (HCT) is a potentially
curative therapy for a variety of malignant and nonmalignant hematological diseases (Thomas et al. 1999; Atkinson 2000). Conventional
HCT is composed of three major components. The first is the administration of marrow ablative conditioning regimens which may consist
of high-dose chemotherapy with or without maximally tolerated doses
of total body irradiation (TBI) and are aimed at both eradicating underlying diseases and suppressing the hosts' immune systems to accept
the allografts. The second is infusion of the allografts to rescue patients from the lethal marrow toxicity of the conditioning regimens.
The third consists of postgrafting immunosuppression or T-cell depletion of the grafts to control graft-versus-host disease (GVHD). Conditioning regimens for conventional HCT have been intensified to the
limits of organ tolerance in order to optimize disease eradication. Consequently, serious toxicities to organs such as gut, lung, kidney, heart,
and liver have been observed which, additionally, have limited the
ability to deliver adequate doses of postgrafting immunosuppression
needed for control of GVHD. Also, myeloablation and immunosuppression caused by the conditioning regimens set the stage for serious
infections. These toxicities have limited conventional HCT to relatively young patients who are in good medical condition. As a result, very
few patients older than 50 years and virtually none older than 60 years
have been treated by allogeneic HCT (Molina and Storb 2000). This
age restriction is unfortunate since the median ages of patients with
most candidate diseases for HCT, e.g., acute and chronic leukemias,
myelodysplasia (MDS), multiple myeloma (MM), and lymphomas,
range from 65 to 70 years (Table 1). Also, in many cases medical comorbidities precluded treatment with allogeneic HCT even in younger
patients (Thomas et al. 1999; Atkinson 2000).
    Early in the history of HCT, it became apparent that even the
most intense conditioning regimens may not be able to eradicate all
hematological malignancies (Thomas et al. 1975). As early as 1979,
graft-versus-tumor (GVT) effects via donor T cells were described
as being as or even more powerful than the conditioning regimens in
controlling and preventing disease recurrence after allogeneic HCT
(Weiden et al. 1979, 1981 a, b; Horowitz et al. 1990).

Table 1. Patient ages at diagnoses and at HCT (Molina and Storb 2000)

	Median patient ages (years)		
	Recent allogeneic HCT recipients (FHCRC)		At diagnosis
Disease	Related donor	Unrelated donor	(SEERS)
CML	40	36	67
AML	28	33	68
NHL	33	35	65
MM	45	45	70
CLL	51	46	71
HD	29	28	34
MDS	40	41	68
Overall	40 ($n = 1428$)	35 ($n = 1277$)	

HSCT, hematopoietic stem cell transplantation; FHCRC, Fred Hutchinson Cancer Research Center; SEERS, Surveillance, Epidemiology and End Results; CML, chronic myeloid leukemia; AML, acute myeloid leukemia; NHL, non-Hodgkin's lymphoma; MM, multiple myeloma; CLL, chronic lymphocytic leukemia; HD, Hodgkin's disease; MDS, myelodysplastic syndrome.

Given the limiting toxicities of conventional conditioning regimens and the observed powerful GVT effects, a number of investigators have developed reduced-intensity conditioning regimens that are less toxic and rely more heavily on GVT effects for gradual disease eradication. The Seattle group, with the help of preclinical studies in a canine model, developed a truly nonmyeloablative conditioning regimen with acceptable toxicities suitable for elderly and/or medically unfit patients who previously were ineligible for HCT.

10.2 GVT Effect

As early as 1956, Barnes et al. using a murine model of leukemia, concluded that high-dose conditioning regimens alone were inadequate to completely eradicate all cancer cells and that the antitumor effect of hematopoietic cell allografts contributed to cure of malignancy (Barnes et al. 1956). Burchenal et al. showed that extremely

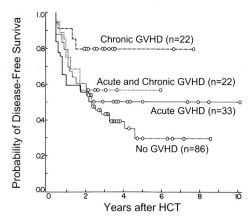

Fig. 1. Disease-free survivals of patients with hematological malignancies given cyclophosphamide and TBI, HLA-matched related HCT, and MTX for GVHD prevention. Shown are data in patients with and without acute and chronic GVHD. (From Weiden et al. 1981 c)

high doses of TBI, far higher than those tolerated by human patients, were needed to kill the last tumor cells in a murine leukemia model (Burchenal et al. 1960). In 1965, Mathé et al. coined the term adoptive immunotherapy to describe this phenomenon (Mathé et al. 1965). In 1979 and 1981, the Seattle transplant team provided practical proof for Mathé's hypothesis by showing that the probability of leukemic relapse was significantly less in patients with acute or chronic GVHD compared to patients without GVHD and those with syngeneic donors (Fig. 1; Weiden et al. 1979, 1981 c). These observations were subsequently confirmed by others (Sullivan et al. 1989; Horowitz et al. 1990). The important roles of T-cells in securing engraftment and effecting GVT effects were illustrated by findings in patients given T-cell-depleted grafts (Martin et al. 1985; Goldman et al. 1988; Gale et al. 1989; Marmont et al. 1991). These patients had less GVHD, but higher rates of graft rejection and disease relapse. Further evidence for a role of donor T-cells in controlling leukemia came from observations by Kolb et al., who induced cytogenetic remissions in three patients with relapsed chronic myeloid leukemia (CML) after allogeneic HCT by using donor lymphocytes infusions (DLI; Kolb et al. 1990). Others confirmed the effectiveness of DLI in larger numbers of patients (Kolb et al. 1995; Slavin et al. 1995; Collins et al. 2000). GVT reactions were presumed to be directed at polymorphic minor histocompatibility antigens including hematopoietic antigens on normal and malignant marrow cells (reviewed in Goulmy 1997; Riddell and Greenberg 1999). Efforts are under way to better define those polymorphic minor antigens and establish more effective adoptive immunotherapy.

10.3 Preclinical Data from a Canine Model

Principles obtained from studies of HCT in random bred dogs have been successfully translated to the setting of human patients. Canine studies have also formed the basis for some of the clinical investigations on nonmyeloablative conditioning regimens.

10.3.1 Development of the Nonmyeloablative Conditioning

10.3.1.1 Concept
The concept of nonmyeloablative conditioning was based on two facts and two hypotheses. The two facts were that T-cells mediate both host-versus-graft (HVG) and GVH reactions after HCT in the major histocompatibility complex-identical setting. The first hypothesis was that the HVG reaction could be controlled by the same immunosuppressive agents that were used to alleviate GVHD. A second hypothesis was that allografts could create their own marrow spaces through GVH reactions. Consequently, we speculated that much of the toxic and myeloablative conditioning could be effectively replaced by optimal posttransplant immunosuppression.

10.3.1.2 Doses of TBI Needed for Dog Leukocyte Antigen-Identical Marrow Engraftment Without Postgrafting Immunosuppression
Using gradually de-escalated single doses of TBI to condition dogs for dog leukocyte antigen (DLA)-identical marrow grafts, we found that graft rejections increased in inverse proportions to the TBI doses used (Storb et al. 1989). After a single dose of 920 cGy, 95% of dogs showed sustained engraftment in the absence of postgrafting

Table 2. TBI doses required for engraftment of DLA-identical marrow without postgrafting immunosuppression

Doses of TBI (cGy)[a]	Dogs studied (n)	Sustained engraftment (%)	Autologous recovery (%)
920 Immunosuppressive	21	95	0
800	5	80	0
700	5	60	0
600	23	52	17
450 Myeloablative and supralethal	39	41	36

[a] Delivered at 7 cGy/min from two opposing [60]Cobalt sources.

Table 3. Marrow toxicity of TBI in dogs not rescued by subsequent HCT grafts

Single dose of TBI (cGy)[a]	Surviving dogs (n)/dogs studied (n)
400 Myeloablative and supralethal	1/28
300	7/21
200 Sublethal	17/18
100	12/12

[a] Delivered at 10 or 7 cGy/min from two opposing [60]Cobalt sources.

immunosuppression while after a dose of 450 cGy, which was still myeloablative and supralethal, only 41% of dogs achieved sustained engraftment; the remainder experienced graft rejection and either died from marrow aplasia (23%) or survived with autologous marrow recovery (36%; Table 2).

10.3.1.3 TBI Marrow Toxicity

In order to define lethal and sublethal TBI doses, de-escalating radiation doses were given to dogs under intensive supportive care, but without rescue by HCT. Only 1 of 28 dogs survived after 400 cGy TBI. In contrast, 200 cGy were found sublethal with 17 of 18 dogs surviving with spontaneous hematopoietic recovery (Table 3). After 200 cGy TBI, a median granulocyte nadir of 750/μl was reached by day 20 before recovery, which was complete by day 40. The median platelet nadir of 7,500/μl was reached between days 15 and 24 before recovery, which was complete by day 50.

10.3.1.4 Engraftment and Mixed Chimerism Using Low-Dose TBI and Postgrafting Immunosuppression

A first study evaluated the usefulness of postgrafting immunosuppression after DLA-identical marrow grafts in dogs conditioned with 450 cGy TBI (Yu et al. 1995). Three groups of dogs were studied (Table 4). High-dose steroids, previously used by other investigators in human patients (Kernan et al. 1989), were given from day –5 to day 32 to five dogs. All five rejected their grafts; three died from marrow aplasia and two survived with autologous marrow recovery. Next, cyclosporine (CSP) 10 mg/kg bid was given from day –6 to –1 to nine dogs. All nine rejected their allografts, with six dying early and three surviving with endogenous marrow recovery. In contrast, all seven dogs given CSP at 15 mg/kg twice daily (bid) from day –1 to day 35 had sustained grafts. Two of the dogs had mixed chimerism and five converted to full donor chimerism. None of the seven developed GVHD. This experiment provided proof for the ability of postgrafting immunosuppression to control both GVH and HVG reactions. Since similar engraftments rates in dogs not given immunosuppression were only achieved using 920 cGy TBI conditioning, the effect of postgrafting CSP could be equated to 470 cGy TBI conditioning.

Subsequent studies extended the initial observations and asked whether sustained hematopoietic grafts from DLA-identical littermates could be achieved after a sublethal TBI dose of 200 cGy (Storb et al. 1997; Table 5). CSP alone was ineffective in establishing sustained engraftment and all four dogs rejected their allografts after 4 weeks but survived with autologous marrow recovery. In six dogs, methotrexate (MTX) at a dose of 0.4 mg/kg per day on days 1, 3, 6, and 11 was added to CSP; these two drugs have previously been shown to be effective in controlling acute GVHD in dogs and humans (Deeg et al. 1982; Storb et al. 1986). Two of five evaluable dogs achieved stable mixed chimerism and three rejected their allografts. We had previously shown that the combination of CSP and mycophenolate mofetil (MMF) was highly synergistic for GVHD control (Yu et al. 1998). Twelve dogs were given 200 cGy TBI be-

Table 4. Results in dogs receiving 450 cGy and marrow grafts from DLA-identical littermates with or without additional immunosuppression

Group no.	Additional immunosuppression	No. of dogs			Surviving	Successful allograft	
		Studied	Rejection	Early death from aplasia	Autologous recovery	Mixed chimerism	All donor cells
1	Corticosteroids[a]	5	5	3	2	0	0
2	CSP pretransplant[b]	9	9	6	3	0	0
3	CSP after transplant[c]	7	0	0	0	2	5
Controls	None	17	11	7	4	3	3

[a] Prednisone, 12.5 mg/kg PO bid on days −5 to −3 with subsequent taper through day 32.
[b] CSP, 20 mg/kg in divided doses from day −6 to −1.
[c] CSP, 15 mg/kg PO bid on days −1 to 35.

Table 5. Marrow grafts from DLA-identical littermates after conditioning with sublethal TBI doses and postgrafting immunosuppression

TBI dose (cGy)	Postgrafting immuno-suppression	No. of dogs Studied	Sustained engraftment	Duration of mixed chimerism (weeks)
200[a]	CSP[b]	4	0	4, 4, 4, 4
200	MTX[c]/CSP[b]	6	3	2, 7, 11, >8[e], >134, >134
200	MMF[d]/CSP[b]	12	11	12, >25, >34, >49, >55, >56, >62, >63, >73, >104, >130, >130
100	MMF[d]/CSP[b]	6	0	3, 3, 10, 10, 10, 12

[a] Delivered at 7 cGy/min.
[b] CSP, 15 mg/kg bid PO on days –1 to 35.
[c] MTX, 0.4 mg/kg IV on days 1, 3, 6, and 11.
[d] MMF, 10 mg/kg bid SC on days 0–27.
[e] Euthanized because of papillomatosis.

fore and MMF, 10 mg/kg bid subcutaneously (SC), on days 0–27 along with CSP after HCT. Sustained mixed chimerism was observed in 11 of the 12 dogs studied with observation periods ranging from 25 to 130 weeks, without GVHD (Storb et al. 1997). However, when the dose of TBI was reduced to 100 cGy, all studied six dogs rejected their allografts after 3–12 weeks.

Surviving stable mixed chimeras were found to have normal immune function as assessed by in vitro lymphocyte responsiveness to alloantigens and concanavalin A, peripheral blood T4/T8 ratios, and humoral antibody responses to sheep red blood cells (Storb et al. 1997). In addition, mixed chimeric dogs accepted skin grafts from their marrow donors, while third party skin grafts were rejected.

Study results confirmed the hypothesis that successful allografts could be achieved by substituting postgrafting immunosuppression for most of the high-dose conditioning regimen.

Mixed donor/host hematopoietic chimerism could be converted into full donor chimerism by infusion of donor lymphocytes that were sensitized to minor histocompatibility antigens of the host

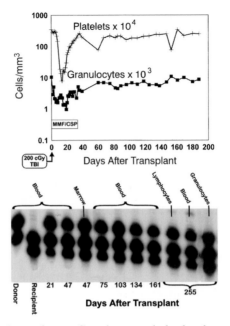

Fig. 2. Sustained engraftment. Granulocyte and platelet changes in dog E131 conditioned with 200 cGy TBI, given a marrow graft from a DLA-identical littermate on day 0 and postgrafting immunosuppression with mycopheno-late mofetil/cyclosporine (*MMF/CSP*) for no more than 35 days. The *bottom panel* shows the results of testing for (CA)$_n$ dinucleotide repeats of donor and recipient cells before transplantation (*lanes 1* and *2*) and recipient cells after marrow transplantation (*lanes 3 to 12*). (From Storb R et al. 1997, with permission)

(Georges et al. 2000; Fig. 2). This finding demonstrated that mixed chimerism established by nonmyeloablative conditioning might be used as a platform for adoptive immunotherapy in patients with hematological malignancies.

In a more recent study, sirolimus (rapamycin) was successfully substituted for MMF. Five of six evaluable dogs given 200 cGy TBI, DLA-identical marrow grafts and a combination of sirolimus and CSP achieved stable mixed hematopoietic chimerism (Hogan et al. 2003).

10.3.2 Defining the Role of Pretransplant TBI: Creation of Marrow Space Versus Host Immunosuppression

In order to distinguish whether the role of 200 cGy was to create marrow space for grafts to home or served to provide host immuno-suppression, the following experiment was carried out. Six dogs were given 450 cGy irradiation restricted to the central cervical, thoracic, and upper abdominal lymph node chain, DLA-identical marrow grafts, and postgrafting MMF/CSP (Storb et al. 1999a). Four of six dogs studied showed sustained engraftment. As early as 6 weeks after HCT, donor cells were found in nonirradiated marrow spaces. Also, donor engraftment was documented in nonirradiated lymph nodes. Dogs had minimal hematological toxicities with plate-let nadirs around 100,000/µl and granulocyte nadirs around 3,000–5,000/µl (Fig. 3). These findings were in keeping with the notion that low-dose TBI provided host immunosuppression and that grafts could create their own marrow space. They raised the possibility that low-dose TBI could be replaced by more specific and less toxic targeted T-cell suppression.

10.3.3 Recent Developments of Targeted T-Cell Therapy

One study explored the use of the fusion peptide CTLA 4Ig, which blocks T-cell costimulation through the B7-CD28 signal pathway. Marrow recipient T cells were activated with intravenous (IV) injec-tions of donor peripheral blood mononuclear cells (PBMC), 1×10^6 cells/kg per day, along with administration of CTLA4Ig, 4 mg/kg per day IV, followed by postgrafting MMF/CSP. All six dogs studied had initial engraftment of DLA-identical marrow and four of the six became stable mixed chimeras (Storb et al. 1999b).

Another study employed a mononuclear antibody to the canine T-cell receptor $\alpha\beta$, which was coupled to a short-lived ($t_{1/2} = 46$ min) α-emitting radionuclide, ^{213}Bismuth (^{213}Bi) (Bethge et al. 2003). All four dogs, given between 3.7 and 5.6 ^{213}Bi mCi/kg before and MMF/CSP after DLA-identical marrow HCT, showed sustained long-term engraftment.

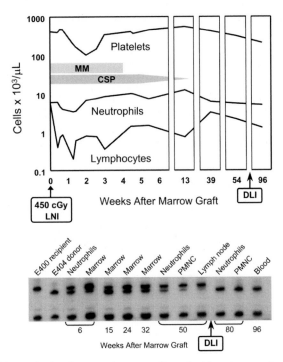

Fig. 3. Hematologic changes (*top panel*) and chimerism analysis results (*bottom panel*) in a dog conditioned with 450 cGy radiation to cervical, thoracic, and upper abdominal lymph nodes before DLA-identical marrow grafts. (From Storb et al. 1999a)

10.4 Clinical Application of Nonmyeloablative Conditioning for HCT

The clinical nonmyeloablative HCT approach was based on the preclinical canine studies. Using this regimen, multicenter studies were conducted by collaborators located at the Fred Hutchinson Cancer Research Center, University of Washington Medical Center, Children's Hospital and Regional Medical Center, and Veterans Administration Medical Center, all in Seattle, WA, United States; Stanford University, Palo Alto, CA, United States; City of Hope National Medical Center, Duarte, CA, United States; University of Leipzig,

Germany; University of Colorado, Denver, CO, United States; University of Torino, Italy; University of Arizona, Tucson, AZ, United States; Baylor University, Dallas, TX, USA; University of Utah, Salt Lake City, UT, United States; Oregon Health Sciences University, Portland, OR, United States; and, more recently, the Medical College of Wisconsin, Milwaukee, WI, United States; and Emory University, Atlanta, GA, United States. Patients on these trials were either elderly or had significant organ comorbidities rendering them ineligible for conventional HCT. Many of them had failed preceding myeloablative autologous or allogeneic HCT.

10.4.1 Initial Clinical Experience with HLA-Matched Sibling HCT

The first clinical study of the nonmyeloablative conditioning included 45 patients with hematological malignancies. The conditioning regimen was identical to that developed in the canine model and consisted of 200 cGy TBI (7 cGy/min) given as a single fraction on day 0, with postgrafting immunosuppression of MMF [15 mg/kg orally (PO) bid from days 0–27] in combination with CSP (6.5 mg/kg PO bid from day −1 to +35 ±taper to day +56; McSweeney et al. 2001). G-PBMC were collected from HLA-identical sibling donors and administered within 4 h of TBI.

The nonmyeloablative regimen was well tolerated. More than half of the eligible patients received their transplants in the outpatient clinical setting. No patient experienced regimen-related painful mucositis, severe nausea and vomiting, pulmonary toxicity, cardiac toxicity, hemorrhagic cystitis, or new-onset alopecia. Mild to moderate nausea and diarrhea due to MMF/CSP were common. Serum creatinine elevations to twice baseline values occurred in 59% of patients because of targeting high serum CSP levels, and resolved in most cases. One MM patient with pre-existing renal dysfunction (serum creatinine 2.3 mg/dl) required hemodialysis. Reversible hyperbilirubinemia to more than 10 mg/dl occurred in three patients because of pre-existing liver cirrhosis, concurrent amphotericin B treatment, and isolated liver GVHD.

All 45 patients had initial engraftment, however nine of them (20%) rejected their grafts after discontinuation of immunosuppression between 2 to 4 months after HCT. Graft rejection was nonfatal in all cases and was followed by autologous hematopoietic recovery similar to the canine observations. Lack of preceding intensive chemotherapy and diagnosis of CML were the main two pretransplant factors predicting graft rejection in this group of patients. Low donor T-cell chimerism at day 28 predicted rejections.

Of 36 patients, 17 (47%) developed acute GVHD, which was grade II in 13 (36%), and grade III in four (11%), and grade IV in none. In most cases, it responded to continuation of CSP and a standard dose of methylprednisolone. Nineteen of 31 evaluable patients developed chronic GVHD requiring systemic immunosuppressive therapy.

Of 36 patients with sustained engraftment, 25 were alive, with 19 (53%) in complete remission (CR), two in partial remission (PR), and four without responses. With a median follow-up of 417 (range 310 to 769) days, 30 of 45 patients (66.7%) were alive. Twelve patients (26.7%) died from disease progression and three from nonrelapse mortality (NRM).

10.4.2 Addition of Fludarabine and Recent Update of Nonmyeloablative HCT from HLA-Matched Related Donors

In order to increase pretransplant host T-cell immunosuppression and prevent graft rejection, Fludarabine at $30 \, mg/m^2/d$ on days -4, -3, and -2 was added to the 200 cGy TBI conditioning regimen (Fig. 4). In yet other patients, mostly with advanced MM, autologous HCT following melphalan was first carried out to decrease the disease burden.

Results, presented at two national meetings, included data from 253 patients with hematological malignancies (including updates on the first 45 reported patients) with a median age of 54 years (range 18–73) (Sandmaier et al. 2001 b, 2002). Of those, 58 patients were conditioned with 200 cGy TBI alone, 118 with fludarabine in addition to TBI (FLU/TBI), and 77 received 200 cGy TBI after cytoreductive autografts (auto/allo). Eighty-eight patients had MM, 40 non-Hodgkin's lymphoma (NHL), 37 MDS/myeloproliferative syndromes (MPS), 27 chronic lymphocytic leukemia (CLL), 24 acute leukemia (AL), 20 CML, and 17 Hodgkin's disease (HD). Transplants were

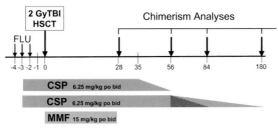

Fludarabine: 30 mg/m^2/day (118 of 253 pts)

Fig. 4. Nonmyeloablative regimen for HCT from HLA-matched related donors

well tolerated with relatively mild hematological changes, and most patients not developing severe neutropenia or thrombocytopenia. Red blood cell and platelet transfusion requirements were significantly lower in recipients of the nonmyeloablative regimen when compared to recipients of conventional HCT (Weissinger et al. 2001). Also, the incidence of cytomegalovirus (CMV) disease was reduced in the first 100 days compared to a matched cohort of recipients of conventional HCT (Junghanss et al. 2002 a), and bacterial infections were significantly less frequent (Junghanss et al. 2002 b).

Median percentages of donor T-cell chimerism on days 28, 56, and 84 were higher among auto/allo and Flu/TBI patients compared to TBI patients ($P \leq 0.005$). Also, graft rejection rates were significantly lower among Flu/TBI (3%) and auto/allo (0%) patients ($P = 0.001$; $P = 0.0001$) compared to TBI patients (17%). Incidences of acute GVHD were comparable between the three patient groups with overall incidences of 31% grade II, 10% grade III, and 5% grade IV in stably engrafted patients. Forty-one percent of patients experienced chronic GVHD.

An increase in NRM was seen among FLU/TBI patients, mainly due to infections and pulmonary events, as compared to TBI patients ($P = 0.02$). Such an increase was not seen among auto/allo patients. With a median follow-up of 387 (range 100 to 1,497) days, the 2-year overall survival (OS) rates were: TBI=55%; FLU/TBI=39%; auto/allo=66%. Potent GVT effects were suggested by the observation of relatively high rates of CR, at the molecular level in patients with CML and CLL, and the morphological level in patients with

AML, ALL, MDS, MM, NHL, and HD. CRs were usually achieved after immunosuppression was tapered and increased donor chimerism was seen. For example, CML patients achieved CR at a median of 5.5 months following HCT (Sandmaier et al. 2001a). Two tentative conclusions were drawn. The first was that cytoreductive autografts before 200 cGy TBI conditioning in patients with NHL and MM were well tolerated and eliminated the risk of graft rejection. The second was that the gain of improved engraftment rates in the FLU/TBI group might be offset by higher rates of NRM leading to lessen OS ($P=0.03$). It followed that the addition of fludarabine should be reserved for patients at high risk for rejection.

10.4.3 Nonmyeloablative Conditioning and HCT with HLA-Matched Unrelated Donors

Encouraged by the success of HCT with HLA-matched related donors, a multi-institutional study of 10/10 HLA-antigen-matched, unrelated donors was initiated in January 2000 (Niederwieser et al. 2003; Maris et al. 2003). Eighty-nine patients were transplanted after conditioning with fludarabine, 30 mg/m^2 per day ×3 days, and 200 cGy TBI. Compared to HLA-matched, related recipients, postgrafting immunosuppression with MMF and CSP was extended to 40 and 100 days, with subsequent tapers to days 96 and 180, respectively (Fig. 5). Donor-recipient matching was done by intermediate resolution DNA typing to a level at least as sensitive as serology for HLA-A, B, and C, and by high-resolution techniques for HLA-DRB1 and DQB1 (Petersdorf et al. 1998). Twenty-one patients had MDS, 12 patients AML, 5 patients ALL, 14 patients CML, 13 patients NHL, 7 patients MPS, 5 patients CLL, 4 patients HD, 7 patients MM, and 1 patient Waldenstrom macroglobulinemia. All patients were ineligible for conventional HCT, 46 because of age, 27 due to failed preceding high-dose HCT, and 16 because of medical comorbidities. Seventy-one patients received G-PBMC and 18 marrow grafts.

   Median patient age was 53 years (range 5–69). Seventy-nine percent of patients showed sustained engraftment while 21% rejected their grafts. In multivariate analysis, graft failure was higher in marrow graft recipients ($P=0.003$) and in those without preceding che-

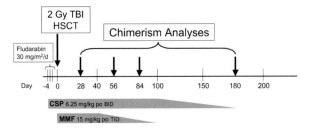

Fig. 5. Nonmyeloablative regimen for HCT from HLA-matched unrelated donors

motherapy ($P=0.003$). Donor T-cell chimerism was higher among G-BPMC recipients compared to marrow recipients at days 28 ($P=0.02$), 56 ($P=0.01$), and 84 ($P=0.08$). Donor T-cell chimerism less than 50% at day 28 predicted graft rejection ($P=0.001$) and relapse ($P=0.05$).

Grades II, III, and IV acute GVHD occurred in 43%, 9%, and 2% of patients with stable engraftment respectively. Chronic GVHD requiring therapy occurred in 40 patients.

Cumulative probabilities of NRM were 11% at day 100 and 16% at 1 year, respectively. With a median follow-up of 13 months (range 5.7–28.4), 42 patients were alive with 69% of them in CR, 12% in PR, and 19% had either stable disease, disease progression, or relapse.

The probability of 1-year OS was 52%, with a trend towards better survival among G-BPMC recipients compared to marrow recipients ($P=0.13$). One-year progression-free survival (PFS) was 38%, with significantly better PFS among G-PBMC compared to marrow recipients (44% versus 17%, $P=0.02$; Fig. 6). Better 1-year PFS and OS rates were observed in patients with B-cell malignancies (53% and 73%, respectively) than in those in patients with AL, CML, or MDS/MPS. While low disease risk, $\leq$5% blasts at time of HCT, female donor, no prior transfusions, and CD3$^+$ cell dose $\geq$ median were all predictive factors for improved OS, the use of G-PBMC and $\leq$5% blasts at time of HCT predicted better PFS.

Given these findings, G-PBMC has become the standard hematopoietic cell source for subsequent unrelated donor nonmyeloablative HCT protocols.

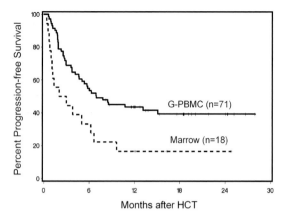

Fig. 6. Kaplan-Meier product estimates of progression-free survival of patients given G-PBMC ($n=71$) or marrow grafts ($n=18$) from HLA-matched unrelated donors. (From Maris et al. 2003, with permission)

10.5 Reduced-Intensity HCT Results from Other Centers

Others have developed reduced-intensity regimens that have retained both substantial antitumor effects and some of the toxicities of high-dose regimens. Typically, combinations of a purine analogue, alkylating agents, and/or monoclonal antibodies were used. Although one of the main aims was to provide sufficient immunosuppression for donor engraftment and subsequent GVT effects, investigators have typically used conditioning agents with wide activities against hematological malignancies in order to prevent tumor progression while awaiting the GVT effects.

10.5.1 M.D. Anderson Cancer Center

Investigators in Houston have explored multiple reduced-intensity regimens that were aimed at tumor-specific cytoreduction of the underlying malignancies. Most of these regimens resulted in successful engraftment with achievement of complete and durable chimerism (Giralt et al. 1997a, b). They used fludarabine/cyclophosphamide and rituximab (anti-CD20 humanized monoclonal antibody) conditioning for HLA-identical sibling HCT, and reported disease-free survival rates of 84% at 2 years in patients with low-grade NHL (Khouri et al. 2001). One report summarized three subsequent trials using different doses of melphalan in combination with fludarabine or cladribine in patients with advanced myeloid leukemia (Giralt et al. 2001). The study showed better engraftment with 2-year OS and PFS rates of 28% and 23%, respectively. However, the melphalan/cladribine arm was closed prematurely because of a high incidence of day-100 NRM (87.5%).

In other studies, 4 patients with MDS and 37 patients with AML were conditioned with fludarabine/busulfan for HCT from related donors, and fludarabine/busulfan/ATG for HCT from unrelated or 1-HLA-antigen-mismatched, related donors. Twenty patients had grade II-III mucositis. One-year OS and PFS were better for patients transplanted in CR (83% and 70%, respectively) than for those transplanted with active disease (30% and 25%, respectively; de Lima et al. 2002).

The fludarabine/melphalan regimen was also used for HCT from either related ($n=13$) or unrelated ($n=9$) donors in 22 patients with MM (Giralt et al. 2002). Seventeen patients engrafted with full donor chimerism, and 7 achieved CR. OS and PFS at 2 years were 30 ±11% and 19±9%, respectively.

Twenty-five patients with advanced HD were conditioned with either fludarabine/melphalan ($n=12$) or fludarabine/cyclophosphamide ±ATG ($n=13$) for HCT from related or unrelated donors. GVHD prophylaxis was tacrolimus and MTX.

Day 30–100 chimerism indicated 100% donor-derived engraftment in the fludarabine/melphalan arm and 58% in the fludarabine/cyclophosphamide ±ATG arm. With a median follow-up of 10 months (1–51), 9 patients died (8 of them in the fludarabine/cyclophosphamide ±ATG arm) and 16 patients (64%) were alive with 9 in remission (Anderlini et al. 2002).

Finally, a retrospective analysis was reported comparing results in 88 patients receiving fully ablative (53 TBI-based and 35 busulfan-based) conditioning and 57 patients receiving fludarabine/melphalan or fludarabine/busulfan reduced-intensity regimens before unrelated donor HCT for treatment of MDS/AML. ATG was added to the preparative regimen in 48% of the cases. At HCT, patients receiving reduced-intensity regimens were significantly older (median age 53 vs. 37 years, $P<0.0001$) and had more primary refractory disease (37% vs. 21%, $P=0.05$) compared to patients receiving fully ablative conditioning. Patients in both groups had similar acute (58% vs. 52%), chronic GVHD (49% vs. 48%) and NRM (51% vs. 46%). The 2-year OS and PFS rates for all patients were 26% and 23%, respectively. Reduced-intensity regimens were not associated with statistically significant survival advantages in univariate or multivariate analyses (Anagnostopoulos et al. 2002).

10.5.2 Hadassah University Hospital

Investigators in Jerusalem developed a conditioning regimen composed of fludarabine (30 mg/m^2×6) and busulfan (8 mg/kg) + peritransplant ATG at 40 mg/kg and postgrafting CSP (Slavin et al. 1998). Twenty-six patients received this regimen followed by HLA-identical sibling HCT, despite absence of clear contraindications for conventional HCT. Median patient age was 31 years (range 1–61). These patients had less advanced diseases than those in the M.D. Anderson studies. Eight patients had CML, six in first chronic phase, one in accelerated phase, and one had juvenile CML. Ten patients had AL, eight in first CR and two in second CR. Two patients had NHL, one had MDS with excess blasts, and one had MM. Four patients had nonmalignant hematological diseases. Patients had high engraftment (100%) and excellent OS (85%) and PFS (81%) rates.

They also reported 100% engraftment rates with this regimen in 23 heavily treated patients with malignant lymphoma (19 had NHL and 4 had HD; Nagler et al. 2000). Seven patients died of NRM and six of relapse. At 37 months OS and PFS were both 40%.

Recently, a good risk group of patients, with CML in first chronic phase and a median age of 35 years, received the same conditioning followed by related ($n=19$) or unrelated ($n=5$) donor HCT. All patients engrafted, with six showing transient mixed chimerism progressing to full donor chimerism. This group of patients showed 0% 100 day NRM with OS and PFS rates of 85±8% (Or et al. 2003).

10.5.3 Universities of Dresden and Berlin, Germany

Investigators at the University of Dresden transplanted 42 patients with hematological malignancies using a regimen similar to that developed in Jerusalem. Fludarabine (30 mg/m^2×5), busulfan (6.6 mg/kg, administered IV), and ATG (10 mg/kg) were followed by unrelated donor HCT and postgrafting immunosuppression composed of either CSP, MTX/CSP, or MMF/CSP (Bornhauser et al. 2001). Twelve patients received HLA-mismatched unrelated donor grafts and nine patients received partially T-cell-depleted grafts (CD34$^+$ selection). Graft failure was observed in 21% of patients with higher incidences in CML patients and recipients of HLA-mismatched grafts. Day 100 NRM was 12%. Fourteen patients died of relapsing disease. The 1-year PFS rate was better among patients with lymphoid malignancies (50%) compared to patients with more advanced hematologic malignancies (20%). Recently, investigators at the University of Berlin used the same conditioning regimen to transplant 30 patients with progressive or relapsing CLL from related ($n=15$) or unrelated ($n=15$) donors. At 2-year follow-up, 11 patients were in CR and another 13 in PR with NRM of 15%. The probability of OS and PFS were 79% and 61%, respectively (Schetelig et al. 2002).

10.5.4 National Institutes of Health

Childs et al. reported full donor chimerism and disease regression in 10/14 patients, with hematological malignancies or renal cell carcinoma, using a conditioning regimen composed of cyclophosphamide (120 mg/kg) and fludarabine (125 mg/m^2) followed by related donor allografts and postgrafting immunosuppression with CSP (Childs et al. 1999). Later, they described the use of this regimen in 19 patients with metastatic renal cell carcinoma refractory to cytokine therapy (Childs et al. 2000). Impressively, ten patients showed regression of their metastatic diseases with three achieving CR and seven showing PR. These results suggested GVT effects against an otherwise incurable solid tumor. Recently, they have shown that pretransplant chemotherapies and increased CD34$^+$ cell doses in the allografts facilitated engraftment in patients with metastatic solid tumors (Carvallo et al. 2004).

10.5.5 Massachusetts General Hospital

In part based on preclinical murine studies (Pelot et al. 1999) and in part based on decades of experience with a similar regimen in patients with aplastic anemia, investigators in Boston have used high-dose cyclophosphamide and peritransplant ATG with or without thymic irradiation for transplanting patients with refractory hematological malignancies with HLA-matched or -mismatched related marrow grafts (Sykes et al. 1999; Spitzer et al. 2000). The regimen was aimed both at tumor cytoreduction and development of mixed chimerism, with or without subsequent DLI. Two of 5 patients receiving HLA-haploidentical HCT showed sustained mixed chimerism and disease responses (Sykes et al. 1999). Using the same regimen with HLA-matched related HCT, 18 of 20 patients showed prolonged mixed chimerism and fourteen patients showed evidence of disease responses. DLI was successful in converting mixed chimerism to full donor chimerism and in optimizing GVT effects. At a median follow-up of 445 days, 52% of the patients were alive with 35% in CR (Spitzer et al. 2000).

In another study, the investigators showed that this regimen was tolerated by patients who failed previous autologous HCT. Nine of 13 patients developed grade II-IV GVHD. The 2-year OS and PFS probabilities were 45% and 37.5%, respectively (Dey et al. 2001).

In a subsequent study with HLA-matched related donor HCT, G-PBMC were substituted for marrow. G-PBMC ensured more rapid and robust T-cell recovery, less transfusion requirements, lower incidence of graft failure, and a higher rate of spontaneous full donor chimerism but with a higher incidence of acute GVHD when compared to marrow allografts (Dey et al. 2002).

In an attempt at overcoming the risk of acute GVHD with HLA-haploidentical HCT, the Boston team explored ex vivo T-cell depletion through $CD34^+$ cell selection of G-PBMC. All 4 studied patients achieved initial mixed chimerism without GVHD; however, all four subsequently lost their grafts. DLI was able to convert host T-cell chimerism to full donor chimerism with grade II GVHD in 1 patient and no GVHD in another (Spitzer et al. 2002).

10.5.6 University College of London, England

Investigators at University College of London have conditioned patients with a combination of fludarabine ($150 \, mg/m^2$), melphalan ($140 \, mg/m^2$), and Campath-^{1}H monoclonal antibody (100 mg) for G-PBMC and marrow transplantation from HLA-identical siblings and HLA-matched and -mismatched unrelated donors (Kottaridis et al. 2000; Chakraverty et al. 2002). Postgrafting immunosuppression included mostly CSP alone, but sometimes MTX was added. Campath-^{1}H is a humanized anti-CD52 monoclonal antibody that depleted T-cells and to a lesser extent natural killer (NK) cells. However, its long half-life and persistence in the circulation at time of the HCT resulted in depletion of T-cells and NK cells in the allografts. Both studies showed very low rates of acute GVHD. NRM was acceptable in both studies with PFS rates of 57% and 67% respectively.

Recently, the investigators updated their results in disease-specific HCT. In 94 patients with NHL, 76% achieved full donor chimerism with 1-year NRM of 17%. PFS and OS rates were 58% and 64%, respectively. Not surprisingly, NRM, PFS, and OS rates were all better in patients with low-grade NHL (8%, 70%, and 80%) compared to those with high-grade NHL (33%, 36%, and 33%; Morris et al. 2002). With a median follow-up of 26 months (range 2–49), the actuarial 4-year OS rate for all patients was 64% with 58% PFS.

Outcomes were less favorable in 27 ALL patients with 2-year NRM and OS rates of 23% and 31%, respectively and 49% of patients showing disease progression (Martino et al. 2003).

Twenty good-risk MM patients received the same regimen followed by related or unrelated donor HCT. NRM was 15% and disease responses were modest with two patients in CR, four in PR, two with minimal responses, six without change, three with progressive disease, and three unevaluable. Consistent with results of past studies of T-cell depletion following myeloablative conditioning, response durations were short (less than 12 months in 5 patients) and late relapses/progressions occurred reflecting delayed immune reconstitution as a consequence of T-cell and NK-cell depletion with Campath-^{1}H. Two-year estimated OS and PFS rates were 71% and 30%, respectively (Peggs et al. 2003).

References

Anagnostopoulos A, de Lima M, Munsell M, Shahjahan M, Couriel D, Martin T, Cano P, McMannis J, Gajewski J, Anderson B, Champlin R, Giralt S (2002) Unrelated donor bone marrow transplantation (UDR) for adults with AML/MDS: similar outcomes with ablative or reduced intensity preparative regimens (RIPR) (abstract). Blood 100 (Part 1):635a, 2502

Anderlini P, Acholonu S, Okoroji GJ, Giralt S, Ueno N, Donato M, Andersson BS, Khouri I, Couriel D, Ippoliti C, Valverde RB, Champlin RE (2002) Reduced early transplant-related mortality following allogeneic stem cell transplantation (SCT) with fludarabine-based, reduced-intensity conditioning from matched related and unrelated donors in advanced Hodgkin's disease (HD) (abstract). Blood 100 (Part 1):620a, 2444

Atkinson K (ed) (2000) Clinical bone marrow and blood stem cell transplantation. Cambridge University Press, Cambridge, UK

Barnes DWH, Corp MJ, Loutit JF, Neal FE (1956) Treatment of murine leukaemia with x-rays and homologous bone marrow. Preliminary communication. Br Med J 2:626–627

Bethge WA, Wilbur DS, Storb R, Hamlin DK, Santos EB, Brechbiel MW, Fisher DR, Sandmaier BM (2003) Selective T-cell ablation with bismuth-213 labeled anti-TCR$\alpha\beta$ as nonmyeloablative conditioning for allogeneic canine marrow transplantation. Blood 101:5068–5075

Bornhauser M, Thiede C, Platzbecker U, Jenke A, Helwig A, Plettig R, Freiberg-Richter J, Rollig C, Geissler G, Lutterbeck K, Oelschlagel U, Ehninger G (2001) Dose-reduced conditioning and allogeneic hematopoietic stem cell transplantation from unrelated donors in 42 patients. Clin Cancer Res 7:2254–2262

Burchenal JH, Oettgen HF, Holmberg EAD, Hemphill SC, Reppert JA (1960) Effect of total body irradiation on the transplantability of mouse leukemias. Cancer Res 20:425–430

Carvallo C, Geller N, Kurlander R, Srinivasan R, Mena O, Igarashi T, Griffith LM, Linehan WM, Childs RW (2004) Prior chemotherapy and allograft CD34$^+$ dose impact donor engraftment following nonmyeloablative allogeneic stem cell transplantation in patients with solid tumors. Blood 103:1560–1563

Chakraverty R, Peggs K, Chopra R, Milligan DW, Kottaridis PD, Verfuerth S, Geary J, Thuraisundaram D, Branson K, Chakrabarti S, Mahendra P, Craddock C, Parker A, Hunter A, Hale G, Waldmann H, Williams CD, Yong K, Linch DC, Goldstone AH, Mackinnon S (2002) Limiting transplantation-related mortality following unrelated donor stem cell transplantation by using a nonmyeloablative conditioning regimen. Blood 99:1071–1078

Childs R, Clave E, Contentin N, Jayasekera D, Hensel N, Leitman S, Read EJ, Carter C, Bahceci E, Young NS, Barrett AJ (1999) Engraftment kinetics after nonmyeloablative allogeneic peripheral blood stem cell transplantation: full donor T-cell chimerism precedes alloimmune responses. Blood 94:3234–3241

Childs R, Chernoff A, Contentin N, Bahceci E, Schrump D, Leitman S, Read EJ, Tisdale J, Dunbar C, Linehan WM, Young NS, Barrett AJ (2000) Regression of metastatic renal-cell carcinoma after nonmyeloablative allogeneic peripheral-blood stem-cell transplantation. N Engl J Med 343:750–758

Collins RH Jr, Goldstein S, Giralt S, Levine J, Porter D, Drobyski W, Barrett J, Johnson M, Kirk A, Horowitz M, Parker P (2000) Donor leukocyte infusions in acute lymphocytic leukemia. Bone Marrow Transplant 26:511–516

de Lima M, Couriel D, Shahjahan M, Madden T, Gajewski J, Giralt S, Russell J, Champlin RE, Andersson BS (2002) Allogeneic transplantation for acute myeloid leukemia (AML) and myelodysplastic syndrome (MDS) using a low-toxicity combination of intravenous (IV) busulfan (Bu) and fludarabine (Flu) + ATG (abstract). Blood 100 (Part 1):853a, #3366

Deeg HJ, Storb R, Weiden PL, Raff RF, Sale GE, Atkinson K, Graham TC, Thomas ED (1982) Cyclosporin A and methotrexate in canine marrow transplantation: engraftment, graft-versus-host disease, and induction of tolerance. Transplantation 34:30–35

Dey BR, McAfee S, Sackstein R, Colby C, Saidman S, Weymouth D, Poliquin C, Vanderklish J, Sachs DH, Sykes M, Spitzer TR (2001) Successful allogeneic stem cell transplantation with nonmyeloablative conditioning in patients with relapsed hematologic malignancy following autologous stem cell transplantation. Biol Blood Marrow Transplant 7:604–612

Dey BR, McAfee SL, Colby C, Sackstein R, Saidman S, Tarbell N, Sachs DH, Sykes M, Spitzer TR (2002) Comparison of outcomes after transplantation of peripheral blood stem cells (PBSCT) versus bone marrow (BMT) following an identical non-myeloablative conditioning regimen (abstract). Blood 100 (Part 1):424a, #1641

Gale RP, Marmont A, Horowitz M, Bortin MM (1989) T cell depletion to prevent GvHD: preliminary univariate analyses of the IBMTR. Bone Marrow Transplant 4(Suppl 2):121

Georges GE, Storb R, Thompson JD, Yu C, Gooley T, Bruno B, Nash RA (2000) Adoptive immunotherapy in canine mixed chimeras after nonmyeloablative hematopoietic cell transplantation. Blood 95:3262–3269

Giralt S, Estey E, Albitar M, van Besien K, Rondón G, Anderlini P, O'Brien S, Khouri I, Gajewski J, Mehra R, Claxton D, Andersson B, Beran M, Przepiorka D, Koller C, Kornblau S, Körbling M, Keating M, Kantarjian H, Champlin R (1997a) Engraftment of allogeneic hematopoietic progenitor cells with purine analog-containing chemotherapy: harnessing graft-versus-leukemia without myeloablative therapy. Blood 89:4531–4536

Giralt S, Gajewski J, Khouri I, Korbling M, Claxton D, Mehra R, Przepiorka D, Andersson B, Talpaz M, Kantarjian H, Champlin R (1997b) Induction of graft-vs-leukemia (GVL) as primary treatment of chronic myelogenous leukemia (CML) (abstract). Blood 90 (Part 1):418a, #1857

Giralt S, Thall PF, Khouri I, Wang X, Braunschweig I, Ippolitti C, Claxton D, Donato M, Bruton J, Cohen A, Davis M, Andersson BS, Anderlini P, Gajewski J, Kornblau S, Andreeff M, Przpiorka D, Ueno NT, Molldrem J, Champlin R (2001) Melphalan and purine analog-containing preparative regimens: reduced-intensity conditioning for patients with hematologic malignancies undergoing allogeneic progenitor cell transplantation. Blood 97:631–637

Giralt S, Aleman A, Anagnostopoulos A, Weber D, Khouri I, Anderlini P, Molldrem J, Ueno NT, Donato M, Korbling M, Gajewski J, Alexanian R, Champlin R (2002) Fludarabine/melphalan conditioning for allogeneic transplantation in patients with multiple myeloma. Bone Marrow Transplant 30:367–373

Goldman JM, Gale RP, Horowitz MM, Biggs JC, Champlin RE, Gluckman E, Hoffmann RG, Jacobsen SJ, Marmont AM, McGlave PB, Messner HA, Rimm AA, Rozman C, Speck B, Tura S, Weiner RS, Bortin MM (1988) Bone marrow transplantation for chronic myelogenous leukemia in chronic phase: increased risk of relapse associated with T-cell depletion. Ann Intern Med 108:806–814

Goulmy E (1997) Human minor histocompatibility antigens: new concepts for marrow transplantation and adoptive immunotherapy (review). Immunol Rev 157:125–140

Hogan WJ, Little M-T, Zellmer E, Friedetzky A, Diaconescu R, Gisburne S, Lee R, Kuhr C, Storb R (2003) Postgrafting immunosuppression with sirolimus and cyclosporine facilitates stable mixed hematopoietic chimerism in dogs given sublethal total body irradiation before marrow transplantation from DLA-identical littermates. Biol Blood Marrow Transplant 9:489–495

Horowitz MM, Gale RP, Sondel PM, Goldman JM, Kersey J, Kolb H-J, Rimm AA, Ringden O, Rozman C, Speck B, Truitt RL, Zwaan FE, Bortin MM (1990) Graft-versus-leukemia reactions after bone marrow transplantation. Blood 75:555–562

Junghanss C, Boeckh M, Carter RA, Sandmaier BM, Maris MB, Maloney DG, Chauncey T, McSweeney PA, Little M-T, Corey L, Storb R (2002a) Incidence and outcome of cytomegalovirus infections following nonmyeloablative compared with myeloablative allogeneic stem cell transplantation, a matched control study. Blood 99:1978–1985

Junghanss C, Marr KA, Carter RA, Sandmaier BM, Maris MB, Maloney DG, Chauncey T, McSweeney PA, Storb R (2002b) Incidence and outcome of bacterial and fungal infections following nonmyeloablative compared with myeloablative allogeneic hematopoietic stem cell transplantation: a matched control study. Biol Blood Marrow Transplant 8:512–520

Kernan NA, Bordignon C, Heller G, Cunningham I, Castro-Malaspina H, Shank B, Flomenberg N, Burns J, Yang SY, Black P, Collins NH, O'Reilly RJ (1989) Graft failure after T-cell-depleted human leukocyte antigen identical marrow transplants for leukemia: I. Analysis of risk factors and results of secondary transplants. Blood 74:2227–2236

Khouri IF, Saliba RM, Giralt SA, Lee M-S, Okoroji G-J, Hagemeister FB, Korbling M, Younes A, Ippoliti C, Gajewski JL, McLaughlin P, Anderlini P, Donato ML, Cabanillas FF, Champlin RE (2001) Nonablative allogeneic hematopoietic transplantation as adoptive immunotherapy for indolent lymphoma: low incidence of toxicity, acute graft-versus-host disease, and treatment-related mortality. Blood 98:3595–3599

Kolb HJ, Mittermüller J, Clemm Ch, Holler G, Ledderose G, Brehm G, Heim M, Wilmanns W (1990) Donor leukocyte transfusions for treatment of recurrent chronic myelogenous leukemia in marrow transplant patients. Blood 76:2462–2465

Kolb HJ, Schattenberg A, Goldman JM, Hertenstein B, Jacobsen N, Arcese W, Ljungman P, Ferrant A, Verdonck L, Niederwieser D, van Rhee F, Mittermüller J, De Witte T, Holler E, Ansari H (1995) Graft-versus-leukemia effect of donor lymphocyte transfusions in marrow grafted patients. European Group for Blood and Marrow Transplantation Working Party Chronic Leukemia. Blood 86:2041–2050

Kottaridis PD, Milligan DW, Chopra R, Chakraverty RK, Chakrabarti S, Robinson S, Peggs K, Verfueth S, Pettengell R, Marsh JCW, Schey S, Mahendra P, Morgan GJ, Hale G, Waldmann H, Ruiz de Elvira MC, Williams CD, Devereux S, Linch DC, Goldstone AH, Mackinnon S (2000) In vivo CAMPATH-1H prevents graft-versus-host disease following nonmyeloablative stem cell transplantation. Blood 96:2419–2425

Maris MB, Niederwieser D, Sandmaier BM, Storer B, Stuart M, Maloney D, Petersdorf E, McSweeney P, Pulsipher M, Woolfrey A, Chauncey T, Agura E, Heimfeld S, Slattery J, Hegenbart U, Anasetti C, Blume K, Storb R (2003) HLA-matched unrelated donor hematopoietic cell transplantation after nonmyeloablative conditioning for patients with hematologic malignancies. Blood 102(6):2021–2030

Marmont AM, Horowitz MM, Gale RP, Sobocinski K, Ash RC, van Bekkum DW, Champlin RE, Dicke KA, Goldman JM, Good RA, Herzig RH, Hong R, Masaoka T, Rimm AA, Ringden O, Speck B, Weiner RS, Bortin MM (1991) T-cell depletion of HLA-identical transplants in leukemia. Blood 78:2120–2130

Martin PJ, Hansen JA, Buckner CD, Sanders JE, Deeg HJ, Stewart P, Appelbaum FR, Clift R, Fefer A, Witherspoon RP, Kennedy MS, Sullivan KM, Flournoy N, Storb R, Thomas ED (1985) Effects of in vitro depletion of T cells in HLA-identical allogeneic marrow grafts. Blood 66:664–672

Martino R, Giralt S, Caballero MD, Mackinnon S, Corradini P, Fernandez-Aviles F, San Miguel J, Sierra J (2003) Allogeneic hematopoietic stem cell transplantation with reduced-intensity conditioning in acute lymphoblastic leukemia: a feasibility study. Haematologica 88:555–560

Mathé G, Amiel JL, Schwarzenberg L, Catton A, Schneider M (1965) Adoptive immunotherapy of acute leukemia: experimental and clinical results. Cancer Res 25:1525–1531

McSweeney PA, Niederwieser D, Shizuru JA, Sandmaier BM, Molina AJ, Maloney DG, Chauncey TR, Gooley TA, Hegenbart U, Nash RA, Radich J, Wagner JL, Minor S, Appelbaum FR, Bensinger WI, Bryant E, Flowers MED, Georges GE, Grumet FC, Kiem H-P, Torok-Storb B, Yu C, Blume KG, Storb RF (2001) Hematopoietic cell transplantation in older patients with hematologic malignancies: replacing high-dose cytotoxic therapy with graft-versus-tumor effects. Blood 97:3390–3400

Molina AJ, Storb RF (2000) Hematopoietic stem cell transplantation in older adults. In: Rowe JM, Lazarus HM, Carella AM (eds) Handbook of bone marrow transplantation. Martin Dunitz, London, UK, pp 111–137

Morris E, Thomson K, Craddock C, Milligan D, Smith GM, Parker A, Schey S, Winfield D, Chopra R, Littlewood T, Tighe J, Hunter A, Kyriakou C, Kottaridis P, Peggs K, Linch D, Goldstone A, Mackinnon S (2002) Long-term follow-up of an alemtuzumab (CAMPATH-1H)-containing reduced intensity allogeneic transplant regimen for non-Hodgkin's lymphoma (NHL) (abstract). Blood 100 (Part 1):40a, #139

Nagler A, Slavin S, Varadi G, Naparstek E, Samuel S, Or R (2000) Allogeneic peripheral blood stem cell transplantation using a fludarabine-based low intensity conditioning regimen for malignant lymphoma. Bone Marrow Transplant 25:1021–1028

Niederwieser D, Maris M, Shizuru JA, Petersdorf E, Hegenbart U, Sandmaier BM, Maloney DG, Storer B, Lange T, Chauncey T, Deininger M, Pönisch W, Anasetti C, Woolfrey A, Little M-T, Blume KG, McSweeney PA, Storb RF (2003) Low-dose total body irradiation (TBI) and fludarabine followed by hematopoietic cell transplantation (HCT) from HLA-matched or mismatched unrelated donors and postgrafting immunosuppression with cyclosporine and mycophenolate mofetil (MMF) can induce durable complete chimerism and sustained remissions in patients with hematological diseases. Blood 101:1620–1629

Or R, Shapira MY, Resnick I, Amar A, Ackerstein A, Samuel S, Aker M, Naparstek E, Nagler A, Slavin S (2003) Nonmyeloablative allogeneic stem cell transplantation for the treatment of chronic myeloid leukemia in first chronic phase. Blood 101:441–445

Peggs KS, Mackinnon S, Williams CD, D'Sa S, Thuraisundaram D, Kyriakou C, Morris EC, Hale G, Waldmann H, Linch DC, Goldstone AH, Yong K (2003) Reduced-intensity transplantation with in vivo T-cell depletion and adjuvant dose-escalating donor lymphocyte infusions for chemotherapy-sensitive myeloma: limited efficacy of graft-versus-tumor activity. Biol Blood Marrow Transplant 9:257–265

Pelot MR, Pearson DA, Swenson K, Zhao G, Sachs J, Yang Y-G, Sykes M (1999) Lymphohematopoietic graft-vs.-host reactions can be induced without graft-vs.-host disease in murine mixed chimeras established with a cyclophosphamide-based nonmyeloablative conditioning regimen. Biol Blood Marrow Transplant 5:133–143

Petersdorf EW, Gooley TA, Anasetti C, Martin PJ, Smith AG, Mickelson EM, Woolfrey AE, Hansen JA (1998) Optimizing outcome after unrelated marrow transplantation by comprehensive matching of HLA class I and II alleles in the donor and recipient. Blood 92:3515–3520

Riddell SR, Greenberg PD (1999) Adoptive immunotherapy with antigen-specific T cells. In: Thomas ED, Blume KG, Forman SJ (eds) Hematopoietic cell transplantation, 2nd edn. Blackwell Science, Boston, pp 327–341

Sandmaier BM, Hegenbart U, Shizuru J, Radich J, Maloney DG, Agura E, Bruno B, Chauncey T, Blume K, Niederwieser D, Storb R (2001 a) Nonmyeloablative hematopoietic stem cell transplantation (HSCT) from HLA-identical siblings for treatment of chronic myelogenous leukemia (CML): induction of molecular remissions (abstract). Blood 98 (Part 2):371 b, #5259

Sandmaier BM, Maloney DG, Gooley T, Hegenbart U, Shizuru J, Sahebi F, Chauncey T, Agura E, Bruno B, McSweeney P, Forman S, Blume K, Niederwieser D, Storb R (2001 b) Nonmyeloablative hematopoietic stem cell transplants (HSCT) from HLA-matched related donors for patients with hematologic malignancies: clinical results of a TBI-based conditioning regimen (abstract). Blood 98 (Part 1):742 a–743 a, #3093

Sandmaier BM, Maloney DG, Gooley TA, Shizuru J, Hegenbart U, Sahebi F, Chauncey T, Bruno B, Agura E, McSweeney P, Forman S, Niederwieser D, Blume K, Storb R (2002) Low dose TBI conditioning for hematopoietic stem cell transplants (HSCT) from HLA-matched related donors for patients with hematologic malignancies: influence of fludarabine or cytoreductive autografts on outcome (abstract). Blood 100 (Part 1):145 a, #544

Schetelig J, Thiede C, Bornhauser M, Schwerdtfeger R, Kiehl M, Beyer J, Kroger N, Hensel M, Scheffold C, Ho AD, Kienast J, Neubauer A, Zander AR, Fauser AA, Ehninger G, Siegert W (2002) Reduced non-relapse mortality after reduced intensity conditioning in advanced chronic lymphocytic leukemia. Ann Hematol 81 (Suppl 2):S47–S48

Slavin S, Naparstek E, Nagler A, Ackerstein A, Kapelushnik J, Or R (1995) Allogeneic cell therapy for relapsed leukemia after bone marrow transplantation with donor peripheral blood lymphocytes. Exp Hematol 23:1553–1562

Slavin S, Nagler A, Naparstek E, Kapelushnik Y, Aker M, Cividalli G, Varadi G, Kirschbaum M, Ackerstein A, Samuel S, Amar A, Brautbar C, Ben-Tal O, Eldor A, Or R (1998) Nonmyeloablative stem cell transplantation and cell therapy as an alternative to conventional bone marrow transplantation with lethal cytoreduction for the treatment of malignant and nonmalignant hematologic diseases. Blood 91:756–763

Spitzer TR, McAfee S, Sackstein R, Colby C, Toh HC, Multani P, Saidman S, Weymouth DW, Preffer F, Poliquin C, Foley A, Cox B, Andrews D, Sachs DH, Sykes M (2000) Intentional induction of mixed chimerism and achievement of antitumor responses after nonmyeloablative conditioning therapy and HLA-matched donor bone marrow transplantation for refractory hematologic malignancies. Biol Blood Marrow Transplantation 6:309–320

Spitzer TR, McAfee SL, Dey BR, Colby C, Hope J, Grossberg H, Preffer F, Saidman S, Shaffer J, Alexander SI, Sachs DH, Sykes M (2002) Ex vivo T-cell depleted non-myeloablative haploidentical transplantation for advanced hematologic malignancy (abstract). Blood 100 (Part 1):638 a, #2513

Storb R, Deeg HJ, Whitehead J, Appelbaum F, Beatty P, Bensinger W, Buckner CD, Clift R, Doney K, Farewell V, Hansen J, Hill R, Lum L, Martin P, McGuffin R, Sanders J, Stewart P, Sullivan K, Witherspoon R, Yee G, Thomas ED (1986) Methotrexate and cyclosporine compared with cyclosporine alone for prophylaxis of acute graft versus host disease after marrow transplantation for leukemia. N Engl J Med 314:729–735

Storb R, Raff RF, Appelbaum FR, Graham TC, Schuening FG, Sale G, Pepe M (1989) Comparison of fractionated to single-dose total body irradiation in conditioning canine littermates for DLA-identical marrow grafts. Blood 74:1139–1143

Storb R, Yu C, Wagner JL, Deeg HJ, Nash RA, Kiem H-P, Leisenring W, Shulman H (1997) Stable mixed hematopoietic chimerism in DLA-identical littermate dogs given sublethal total body irradiation before and pharmacological immunosuppression after marrow transplantation. Blood 89:3048–3054

Storb R, Yu C, Barnett T, Wagner JL, Deeg HJ, Nash RA, Kiem H-P, McSweeney P, Seidel K, Georges G, Zaucha JM (1999 a) Stable mixed hematopoietic chimerism in dog leukocyte antigen-identical littermate dogs given lymph node irradiation before and pharmacologic immunosuppression after marrow transplantation. Blood 94:1131–1136

Storb R, Yu C, Zaucha JM, Deeg HJ, Georges G, Kiem H-P, Nash RA, McSweeney PA, Wagner JL (1999 b) Stable mixed hematopoietic chimerism in dogs given donor antigen, CTLA4Ig, and 100 cGy total body irradiation before and pharmacologic immunosuppression after marrow transplant. Blood 94:2523–2529

Sullivan KM, Weiden PL, Storb R, Witherspoon RP, Fefer A, Fisher L, Buckner CD, Anasetti C, Appelbaum FR, Badger C, Beatty P, Bensinger W, Berenson R, Bigelow C, Cheever MA, Clift R, Deeg HJ, Doney K, Greenberg P, Hansen JA, Hill R, Loughran T, Martin P, Neiman P, Petersen FB, Sanders J, Singer J, Stewart P, Thomas ED (1989) Influence of acute and chronic graft-versus-host disease on relapse and survival after bone marrow transplantation from HLA-identical siblings as treatment of acute and chronic leukemia. Blood 73:1720–1728

Sykes M, Preffer F, McAfee S, Saidman SL, Weymouth D, Andrews DM, Colby C, Sackstein R, Sachs DH, Spitzer TR (1999) Mixed lymphohaemopoietic chimerism and graft-versus-lymphoma effects after non-myeloablative therapy and HLA-mismatched bone-marrow transplantation. Lancet 353:1755–1759

Thomas ED, Storb R, Clift RA, Fefer A, Johnson FL, Neiman PE, Lerner KG, Glucksberg H, Buckner CD (1975) Bone-marrow transplantation. N Engl J Med 292:832–843, 895–902

Thomas ED, Blume KG, Forman SJ (eds) (1999) Hematopoietic cell transplantation, 2nd edn. Blackwell Science, Boston

Weiden PL, Flournoy N, Thomas ED, Prentice R, Fefer A, Buckner CD, Storb R (1979) Antileukemic effect of graft-versus-host disease in human recipients of allogeneic-marrow grafts. N Engl J Med 300:1068–1073

Weiden PL, Flournoy N, Thomas ED, Fefer A, Storb R (1981a) Antitumor effect of marrow transplantation in human recipients of syngeneic or allogeneic grafts. In: Okunewick J, Meredith R (eds) Graft-versus-leukemia in man and animal models. CRC, Boca Raton, pp 11–23

Weiden PL, Storb R, Deeg HJ (1981b) Antitumor effect of marrow transplantation in randomly bred species: studies in dogs with spontaneous lymphoma. In: Okunewick J, Meredith R (eds) Graft-versus-leukemia in man and animal models. CRC, Boca Raton, pp 127–138

Weiden PL, Sullivan KM, Flournoy N, Storb R, Thomas ED, and the Seattle Marrow Transplant Team (1981c) Antileukemic effect of chronic graft-versus-host disease. Contribution to improved survival after allogeneic marrow transplantation. N Engl J Med 304:1529–1533

Weissinger F, Sandmaier BM, Maloney DG, Bensinger WI, Gooley T, Storb R (2001) Decreased transfusion requirements for patients receiving non-myeloablative compared with conventional peripheral blood stem cell transplants from HLA-identical siblings. Blood 98:3584–3588

Yu C, Storb R, Mathey B, Deeg HJ, Schuening FG, Graham TC, Seidel K, Burnett R, Wagner JL, Shulman H, Sandmaier BM (1995) DLA-identical bone marrow grafts after low-dose total body irradiation: effects of high-dose corticosteroids and cyclosporine on engraftment. Blood 86:4376–4381

Yu C, Seidel K, Nash RA, Deeg HJ, Sandmaier BM, Barsoukov A, Santos E, Storb R (1998) Synergism between mycophenolate mofetil and cyclosporine in preventing graft-versus-host disease among lethally irradiated dogs given DLA-nonidentical unrelated marrow grafts. Blood 91:2581–2587

Ernst Schering Research Foundation Workshop

Editors: Günter Stock
Monika Lessl

Supplement 1 (1994): Molecular and Cellular Endocrinology of the Testis
Editors: G. Verhoeven, U.-F. Habenicht

Supplement 2 (1997): Signal Transduction in Testicular Cells
Editors: V. Hansson, F.O. Levy, K. Taskén

Supplement 3 (1998): Testicular Function:
From Gene Expression to Genetic Manipulation
Editors: M. Stefanini, C. Boitani, M. Galdieri, R. Geremia,
F. Palombi

Supplement 4 (2000): Hormone Replacement Therapy
and Osteoporosis
Editors: J. Kato, H. Minaguchi, Y. Nishino

Supplement 5 (1999): Interferon: The Dawn of Recombinant
Protein Drugs
Editors: J. Lindenmann, W.D. Schleuning

Supplement 6 (2000): Testis, Epididymis and Technologies
in the Year 2000
Editors: B. Jégou, C. Pineau, J. Saez

Supplement 7 (2001): New Concepts in Pathology and
Treatment of Autoimmune Disorders
Editors: P. Pozzilli, C. Pozzilli, J.-F. Kapp

Supplement 8 (2001): New Pharmacological Approaches
to Reproductive Health and Healthy Ageing
Editors: W.-K. Raff, M.F. Fathalla, F. Saad

Supplement 9 (2002): Testicular Tangrams
Editors: F.F.G. Rommerts, K.J. Teerds

Supplement 10 (2002): Die Architektur des Lebens
Editors: G. Stock, M. Lessl

Supplement 11 (2005): Regenerative and Cell Therapy
Editors: A. Keating, K. Dicke, N. Gorin, R. Weber, H. Graf

This series will be available on request from
Ernst Schering Research Foundation, 13342 Berlin, Germany